A Book of Yoga

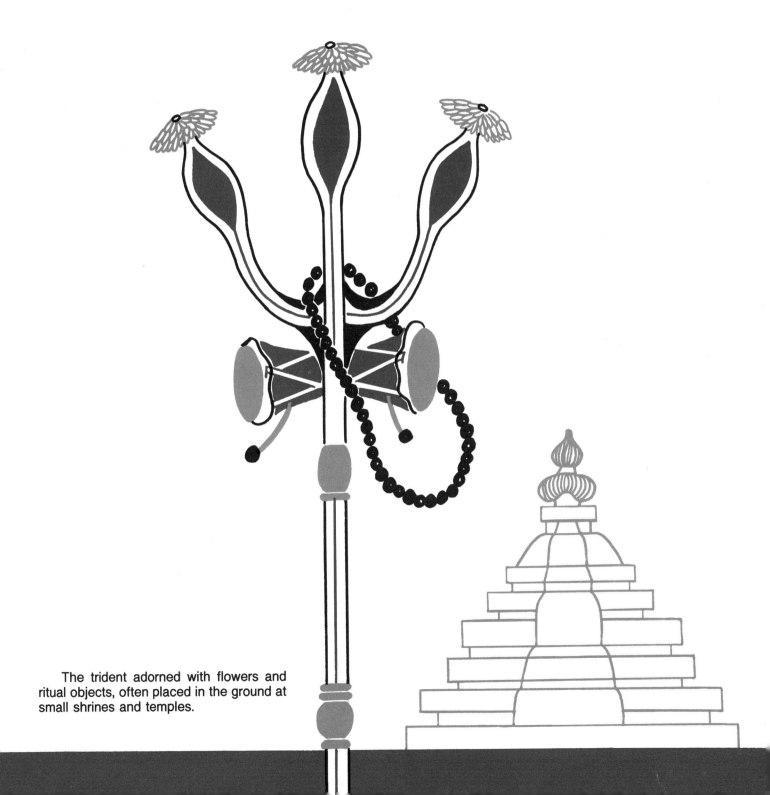

The trident adorned with flowers and ritual objects, often placed in the ground at small shrines and temples.

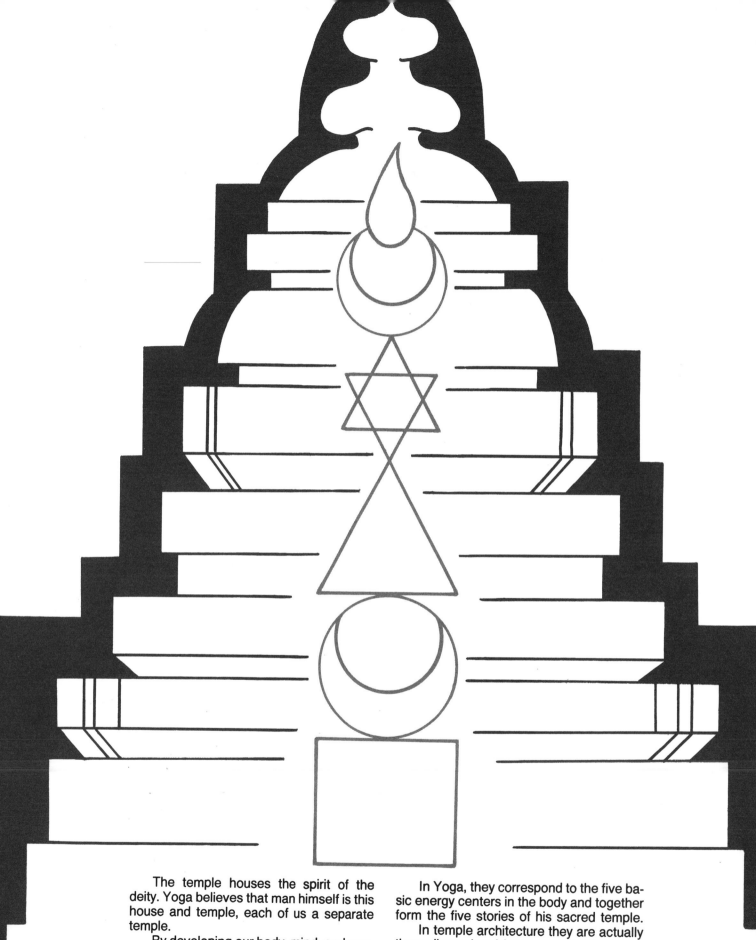

The temple houses the spirit of the deity. Yoga believes that man himself is this house and temple, each of us a separate temple.

By developing our body, mind, and consciousness, we revere the life force in each of us.

The forms for the basic elements in nature, in Eastern symbology, are placed one upon another to make a picture of man.

In Yoga, they correspond to the five basic energy centers in the body and together form the five stories of his sacred temple.

In temple architecture they are actually three dimensional forms used for the base, lower stories, cupola, and upper section of the temple.

On the next page a bas relief from Belur of man as his temple.

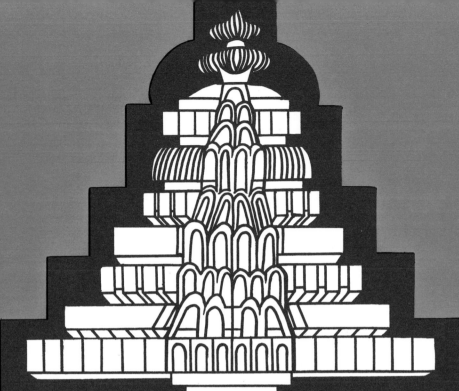
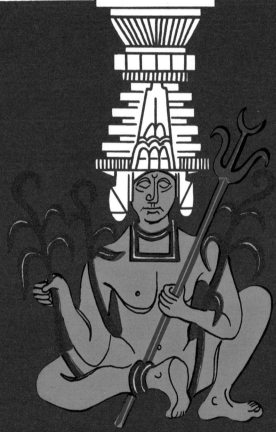

A Book of Yoga
THE BODY TEMPLE

David Weinrib   Jo Ann Weinrib

Photographs by Sandra Hochhausen
Quadrangle/The New York Times Book Co.

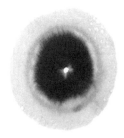

We thank the friends and students we used in the photos—Andre, Charlie, Johanna, John, Mumbie, Robin, and Sheila.

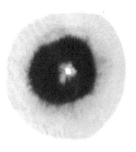

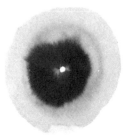

Design Consultant: John Macellari

Library of Congress Cataloging in Publication Data

Weinrib, David.
    The body temple: a book of yoga.

    1. Yoga, Hatha. I. Weinrib, Jo Ann, joint author.
II. Title.
RA781.7.W43 1975   613.7   74-77954
ISBN 0-8129-0494-X

For our first teacher   *For Nina and David*

Our first teacher taught Hatha Yoga in a very alive way, always enriching the teaching of the yoga postures (asanas) with his immense knowledge of medicine, religion and history. He helped toward the inspiration for this book.

We worked with him at an ashram in southern India, studying all aspects of yoga. Near the end of the year's session two other students got together with us to plan some kind of record of the Hatha Yoga postures so that all the students could have a reference after we left. Together we conceived of the prototype for this book. We had the first version mimeographed and then set up a table of paints and colored inks at the ashram so that each student could paint his own book. Our teacher gave his blessing to the project saying, "Yes, that's what yoga books should be like now." We took this to mean that ours was a freer, more colorful, more fluid presentation than that of former yoga books. This of course is in no way intended to diminish the serious books of dedicated masters. This book is just another way of presenting the same timeless material.

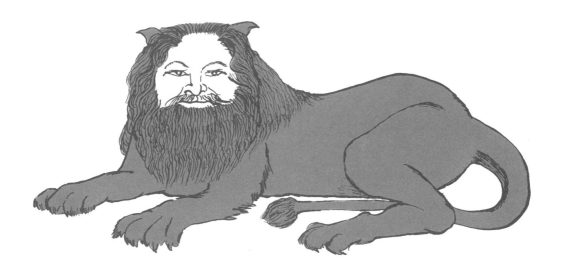

O Ganesha, O Ganesha, may this book spread the living tradition of yoga!

Ganesh, elephant god of the Hindu scriptures, is called upon to remove obstructions that stand in the path of good fortune. Ganesh is the celestial scribe to whom the Bhagavad Gita was dictated. He is invoked at the start of religious ceremonies, births, marriages, and dramatic and literary events.

Hail Ganesha, Hail Ganesha!

Ganesh's father, Shiva, accidentally cut off his son's head and was directed by the gods to replace it with the head of the first being he met, which turned out to be an elephant.

The god Ganesh, in the form of the largest of the earth's land animals, demonstrates his elephantine strength by removing all obstructions; the elephant's amazing memory symbolizes the eternal memory of man.

With his trunk he bellows out the universal OM.

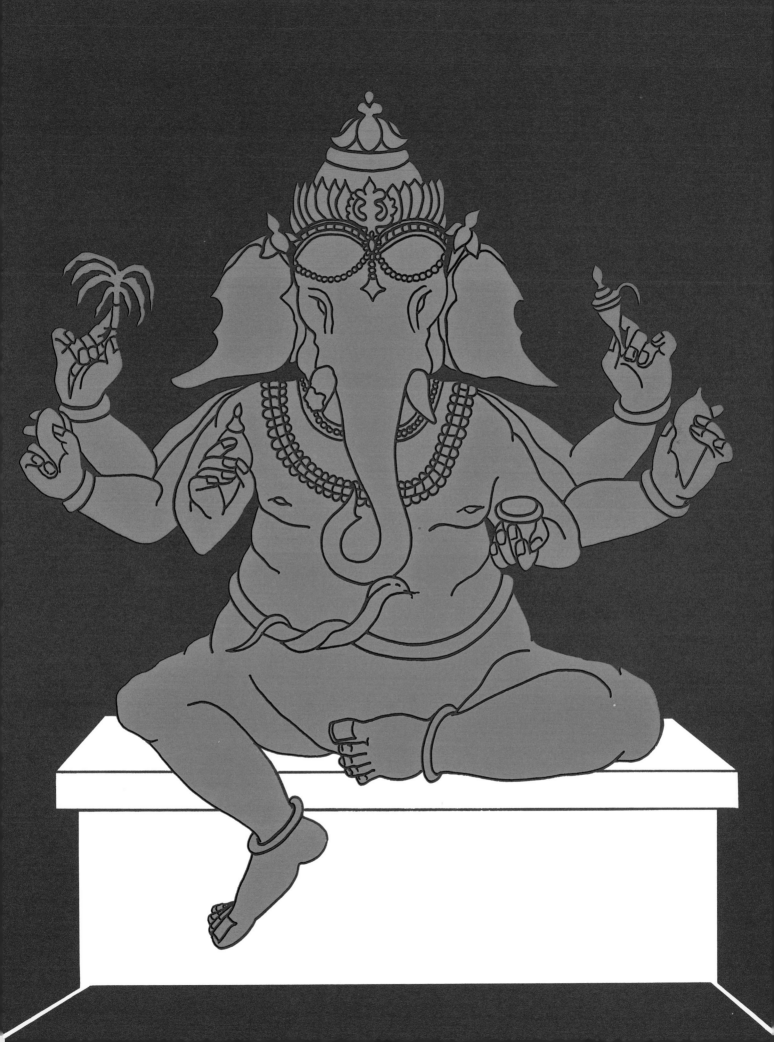

CONTENTS

HATHA YOGA AND THE EIGHT PATHS

There are many paths to a closer unity with the inner spirit–mind. Yoga is all about this union. Its teachings are divided into an eight-part integral system. These parts should not be taken as eight strictly distinct categories. They can lead one to another and intertwine. Different temperaments will often be drawn to different paths. These paths are like the rainbow divisions of the spectrum that are produced when white light passes through a prism.

Hatha Yoga (the yoga of the physical body and the organs within) is the yogic path which leads to dynamic health through the practice of asanas (firm postures), kryas (affecting circulatory activities), and mudras (affecting neuro-muscular activities). The aim of Hatha Yoga is to bring you intimately in touch with your body and its functioning to a point of supersensitivity to its kinetics.

The eight paths shown on the accompanying mandala, moving clockwise from the top, are: HATHA YOGA, KARMA YOGA, the yoga of cause and effect or of selfless service, GNANA YOGA, the yoga of thought and intellect, DHARANA–DHYANA YOGA, the yoga of concentration which leads to meditation, BHAKTI YOGA, the yoga of love and devotion to love, PRANAYAMA YOGA, the yoga of the regulation and control of the breath flow, LAYA YOGA, the yoga of attainment and absorption, and MANTRA YOGA, the yoga of vibration through sound.

Those very advanced in the yoga can watch and control their inner bodily processes. It was through this ability thousands of years ago, before the science of anatomy, before the X-ray, that a group of skilled men were able to probe and develop what can be called the *science* of yoga. Remarkable diagrams and charts have come down to us to illustrate their knowledge—an ancient stone carving still exists showing all the nerve flows in the body. Much of the art of Tantra, on its subtle plane, has to do with the interplay of bodily forces.

The spirit of all the yogas is present in the Hatha Yoga. To move the body in rhythmic ways, to feel the interior fluids flowing, to be conscious of the nerves responding, to feel one posture evolving into the next, to answer the needs of the body in the parts that require revivifying, and to do this in quiet and concentration is a meditation in

itself. It takes much concentration and devotion to pursue this yoga, especially in the kinds of lives most of us live today.

To work with a group can be a great reinforcement, to work with a good teacher is tremendously valuable, but the basic thing that will nurture you is your own enjoyment; the deep joy you feel in the activity of the body, seeing it become more limber, more graceful and in stronger health.

Walk with your back straight and chest out
Supple as a lion
Feel the air move into your lungs
Sense your digestion humming
Feel your skull and brain shining
You are ten feet high
Feel new thoughts and awareness
Feel the beauty of the time of day
When you do your yoga.
Sing, dance, chant,
Feel your new body growing.

We do yoga nude, we do yoga clothed. Much depends on climate and mood. For the book the asanas are often shown in the nude because the body movement is more clearly revealed in this way.

Modern scientific investigators are probing and verifying many of the practices of the different yogas. The direct control of the body by the mind is now being explored in certain therapies dealing with high blood pressure and epilepsy, to enable the patient to control these tendencies.

The connection between body and mind, mind and body, and emotions and physical states was dealt with in these ancient systems as they are in present day psychology and psychosomatic medicine. Yoga can be thought of as a system of preventive medicine.

The healthy body contributes to the healthy mind, the relaxed body contributes to the relaxed mind and emotions.

We must become aware of these connections again and again whenever we lose touch with ourselves.

Exterior treatment, therapies, and drugs (which often take away symptoms but don't cure the illness) all come from outside the body. The more we can train ourselves interiorly—by looking into ourselves more, drawing on ourselves more, being independent and more autonomous—the more we build in new patterns for the entire psyche.

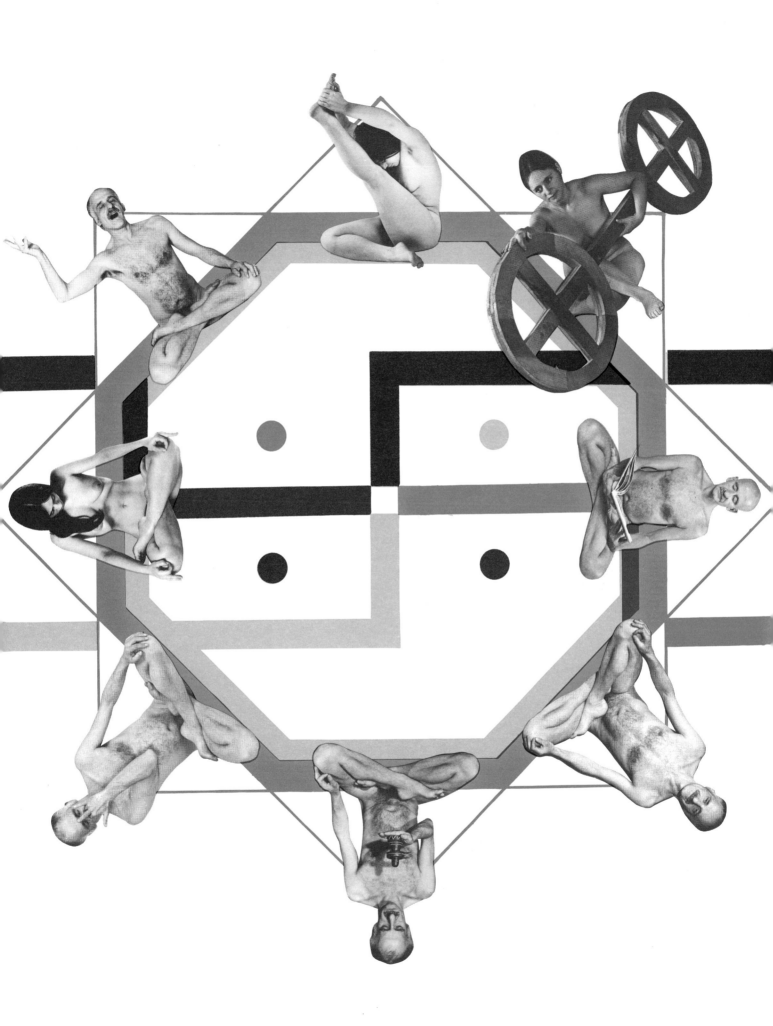

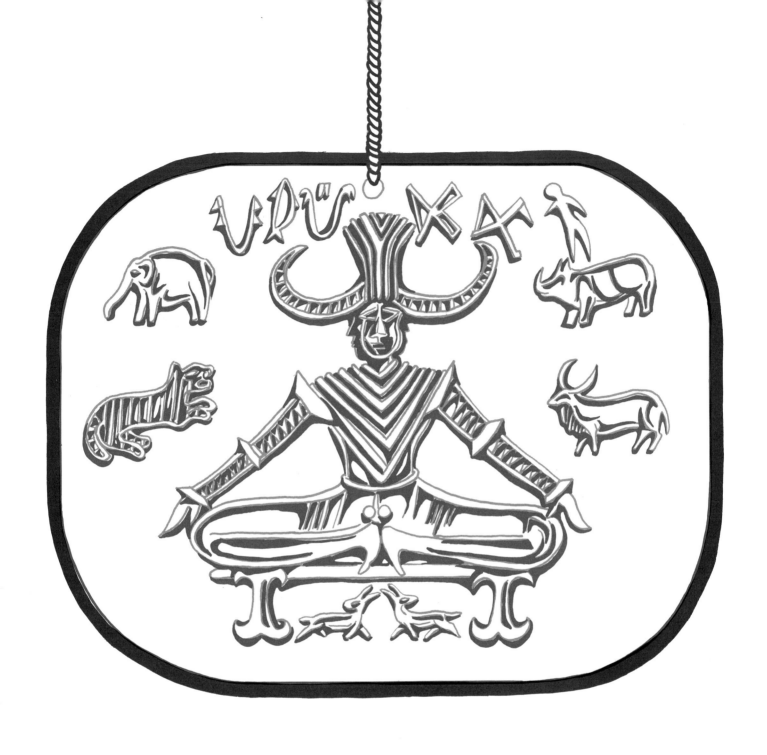

Mohenjo-Daro, Ancient Yoga

A fired clay seal found in the excavations at Mohenjo-Daro, a north Indian civilization whose artifacts date from 2500 B.C.

The first definite historical event in the known record of yoga is the writing of Patanjali circa 200 B.C. It was he who first codified the oral tradition of yogic knowledge.

This clay seal is often pointed to as an indication of how old the knowledge of Hatha Yoga really is.

On it, three faced AM, the supreme god of the ancient Indus valley civilization of northern India, precursor of the Hindu god Shiva, sits in a position called Shakta Chalani.

In a yoga variation on the Shakta Chalani posture, the heel of the foot is put against the vagric nerve that runs very close to the surface between the anus and the sex organs, thus moving sexual energies inwards and upwards. Anthropologists may conjecture whether the figure is truly representative of the Shakta Chalani posture, but it is evident that the feet are in the right area and that the phallus points upward.

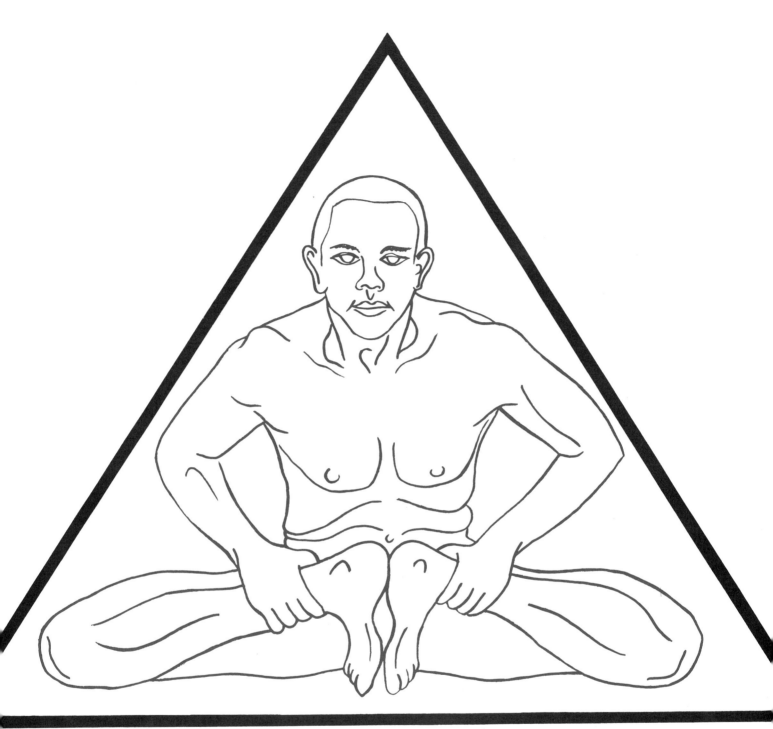

A present day yogi sits in the Shakta Chalani posture.

ANIMAL MOVEMENT IN RELATION TO YOGA

The movements of the jungle animals, carefully observed thousands of years ago, led to the development of many of the positions of Hatha Yoga and a great number of the asanas (postures) are named after them.

The big-cat family was studied in particular. The cat's way of stretching and moving, the graceful succession of extension, holding and release, set the pattern for the yogic rhythm of exercise and control.

Our teacher tells how the ancient yogis learned the nasal douche by observing the elephant and the anal douche by observing the Sarus crane.

Many of the asanas are named after Hindu gods, natural phenomena, birds, fish and insects, and also after symbols and customs in Indian life.

The painting on the next page is of Krishna, one of the Hindu deities in his special form as king of the animals.

In one of the many Hindu stories to illustrate the oneness of all beings, Krishna was asked who he really was. He said he was all of the animals, and in that same instant he changed himself into a collective animal, part cow, part bird, part tiger, part elephant, with the tail of a snake—a representation of all the animals who are symbols of the other gods.

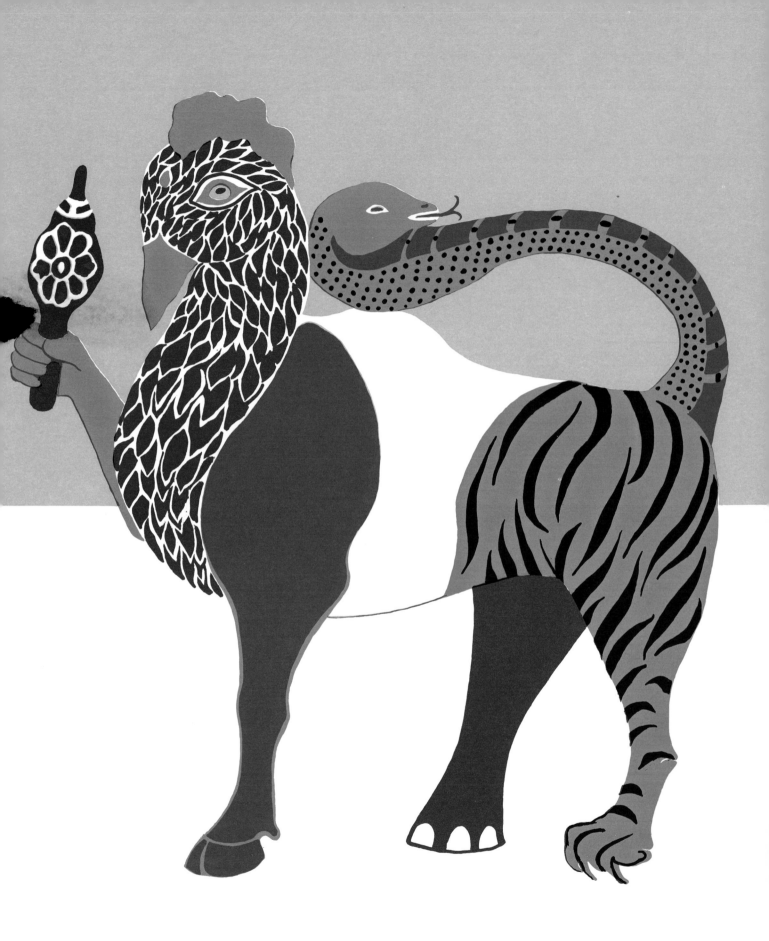

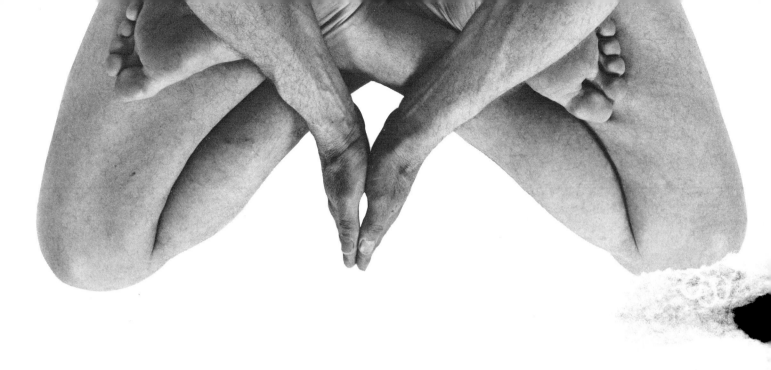

THE FIRST THING

YOU MUST LEARN TO DO IS SIT

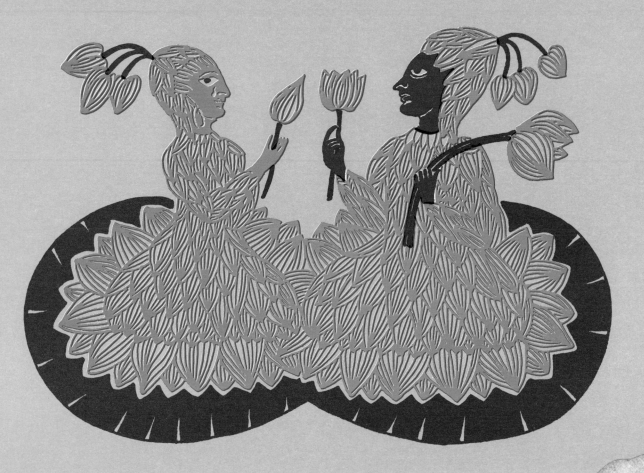

ABOUT SITTING

The first thing you must learn to do is *sit*. Many of us have been trained to sit only in chairs, which were probably invented so that one could get off the cold ground and away from drafts. High backed chairs made a wall against the wind and cold when one faced the fire. Perhaps, too, humans seeking to disassociate themselves from the animal kingdom and nature created furniture. Today, since most of us live in modern buildings with central heating, this way of sitting is not always necessary. Chair sitting does not relax the body. It holds the body with props so that it tends to lose its own strength and resilience.

Sitting on the floor or ground brings one in touch with the base of things. To sit on the ground is to ground yourself physically and psychically, as an electric system is grounded. Sitting on the floor or ground tends to make the body more relaxed and fluid. At first it will be hard for some but if you just start sitting this way whenever you can, old patterns will change; everything in the body will loosen up, and sitting on the floor will become natural again.

In doing yoga one must become relaxed when sitting on the floor, for it is the basis of many of the postures and practices.

Easy Position *Sukasana*

Sit on the floor. Try to keep your back very straight. Your legs are crossed comfortably in front of you. Feel the legs relaxed and spreading. Feel how the spinal column grows from the coccyx and the pelvis like a stamen rising from a blossom.

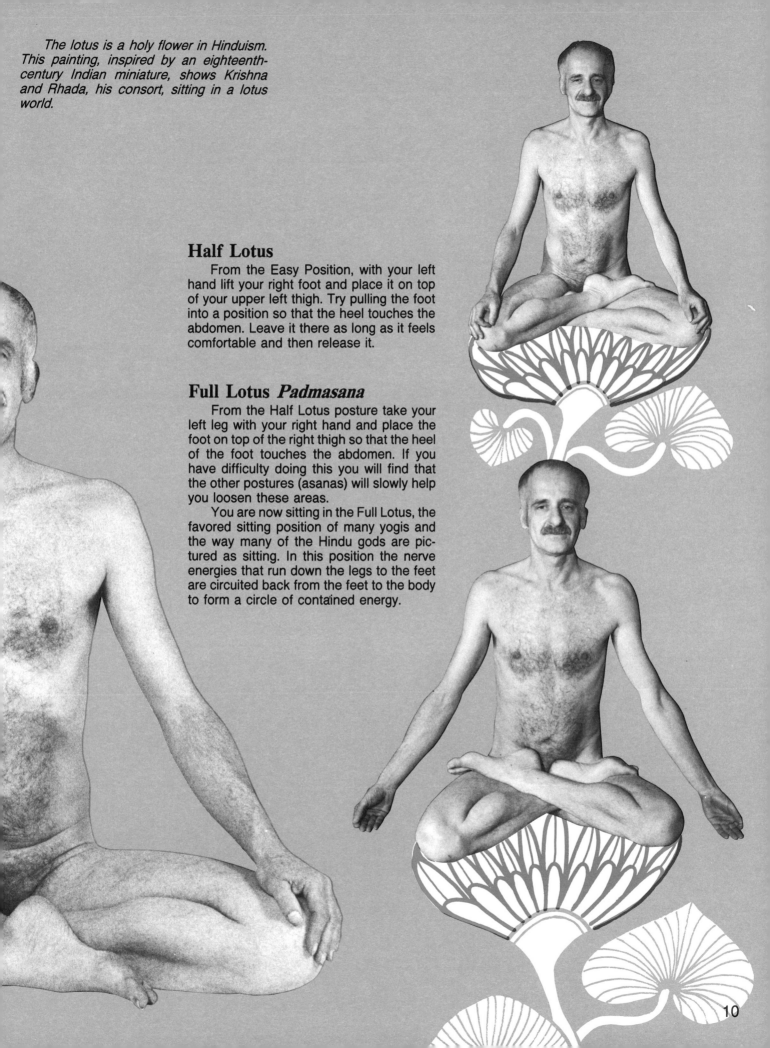

The lotus is a holy flower in Hinduism. This painting, inspired by an eighteenth-century Indian miniature, shows Krishna and Rhada, his consort, sitting in a lotus world.

Half Lotus

From the Easy Position, with your left hand lift your right foot and place it on top of your upper left thigh. Try pulling the foot into a position so that the heel touches the abdomen. Leave it there as long as it feels comfortable and then release it.

Full Lotus *Padmasana*

From the Half Lotus posture take your left leg with your right hand and place the foot on top of the right thigh so that the heel of the foot touches the abdomen. If you have difficulty doing this you will find that the other postures (asanas) will slowly help you loosen these areas.

You are now sitting in the Full Lotus, the favored sitting position of many yogis and the way many of the Hindu gods are pictured as sitting. In this position the nerve energies that run down the legs to the feet are circuited back from the feet to the body to form a circle of contained energy.

10

The dorje or vajra is the Tibetan Buddhist thunderbolt symbol of the thunder god. It is also known as the diamond scepter, the symbol of the highest spiritual power, capable of cutting through any substance.

Indra, the Hindu god of thunder and lightning, rides through the clouds and heavens on his elephant, Airavatam.

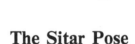

The Sitar Pose

Sit on the floor. Bend your right knee in front of you so that your right foot lies along the left side of the buttocks. Cross the left leg over the right so that the left foot is next to the right thigh and your knees are crossed over one another. This posture is often used in meditation and is a classic pose for Indian instrumentalists.

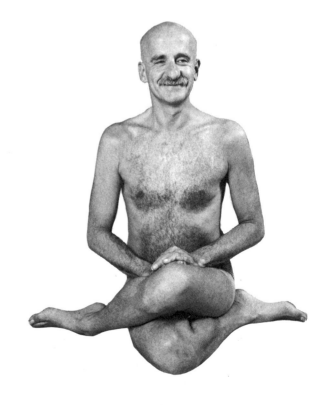

The Thunderbolt *Vajrasana*

Kneel with your feet straight behind you, your heels touching. Your body is in a straight line above your knees. Slowly let your buttocks down so that they rest comfortably on the top of your heels. There should be a straight line from your buttocks to your shoulders and along the back of your head. This is the mighty Thunderbolt pose; the body sits up like a bolt of lighting. This is another pose for meditation, much favored by the Buddhists.

11

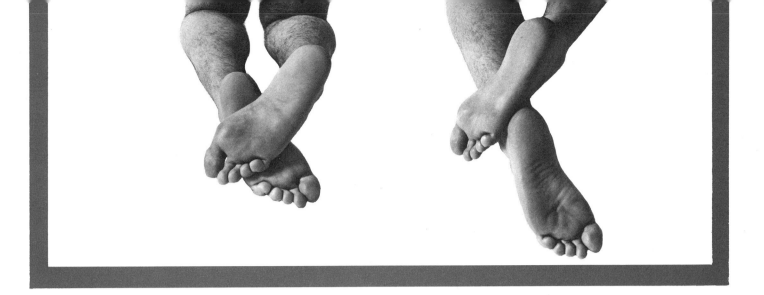

Crossed Heels *Ekakin*

From the Thunderbolt posture raise up on your knees and place one foot inside the instep of the other, and then sit on the heels again. Hold for half a minute. Repeat, reversing the feet. Breathe deeply in this posture. This lockage has a beneficial effect on digestive disturbances besides being good for tired or flat feet.

Spread Heels *Utita*

This is a more relaxed variation to use when you feel strain in the Thunderbolt posture. In this version, the heels are spread rather than close together. For breathing exercises use the more classical pose for you sit more erect.

Locked Heels *Gulpha*

From the Thunderbolt posture raise up on your knees and place one foot over the Achilles tendon of the opposite foot, and then sit on your heels again. Hold for half a minute. Repeat, reversing the feet. This posture stimulates the pituitary and pineal glands, helping glandular troubles in general. The pituitary is the master gland which regulates all the ductless glands in the body. Breathe deeply.

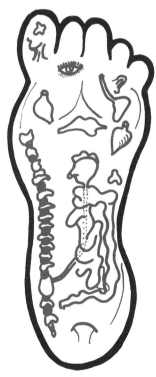

The flat of the foot is a map of the entire body. Nerves from the various parts of the body have endings in different sections of the sole. That is why the above foot postures affect organs and glands. In yoga therapy these sections of the foot are massaged to affect interior parts of the body. This practice finds its present day counterpart in the field of zone therapy.

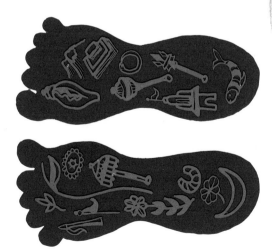

The footprints of the Indian god Vishnu, with symbols and diagrams indicating different aspects of his cosmic nature. On the physical plane, these also could be related to different organs and functions.

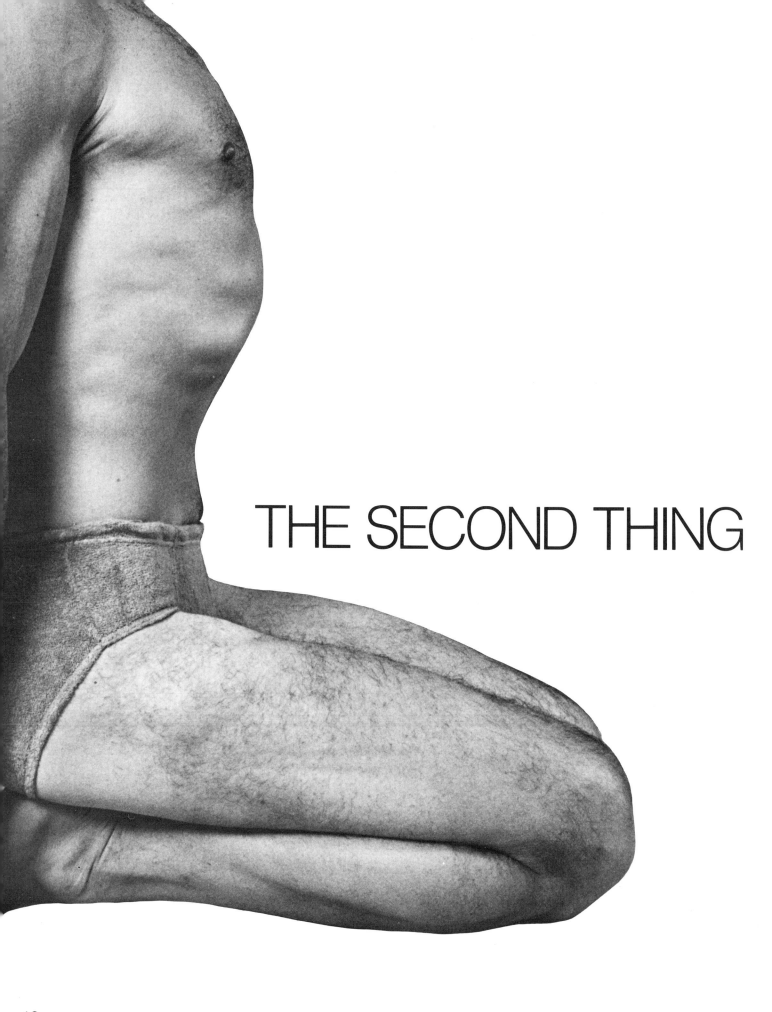

THE SECOND THING

YOU MUST LEARN TO DO
IS BREATHE

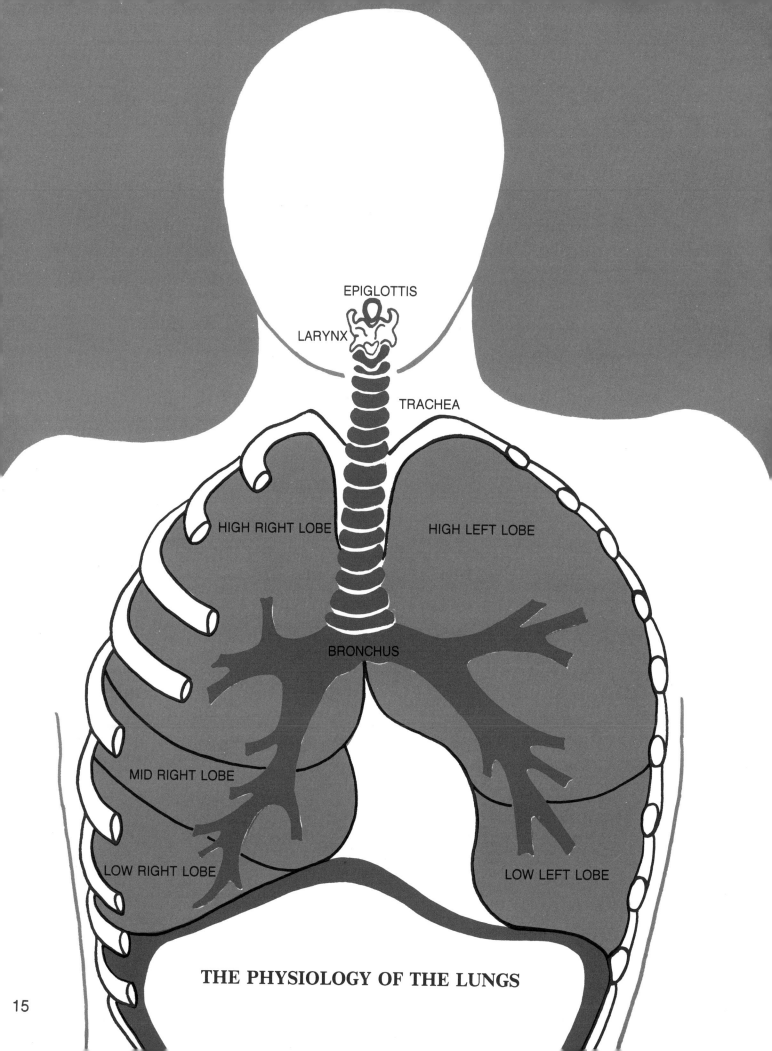

THE PHYSIOLOGY OF THE LUNGS

15

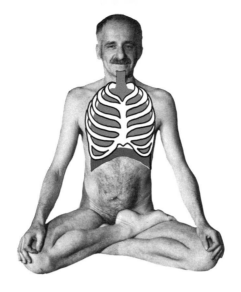

The second thing you must learn to do is breathe.

Close your eyes, take a long deep breath.

Feel where the air is going.

Now, exhale. Try to follow the path of the breath as it leaves the body.

Visualize yourself as a small particle being carried with the air.

The air enters the nose and moves through the coarse hairs of the nasal passage, down along the mucous membrane in the nasal cavities to the back of the skull and into a muscular tube called the pharynx. It passes through the flaplike opening of the epiglottis and into the tunnel of the larynx. Still moving downward, it comes into the extension of the larynx, the trachea, which at its end divides into two branchlike tubes called bronchi. From here the air enters into the spongy cells of the lungs. The lungs expand and contract, filling the entire chest cavity as they do their job of taking in the air and exchanging the gases.

By following this one breath you have gone through the process that, in normal breathing, takes place in your body one thousand times per hour.

The lungs are composed of three lobes on the right side and two front lobes on the left side. (The heart takes up the space that the left middle lobe would occupy.) The air fills the lower lobes in the lower abdominal area, then expands into the mid lobes in the intercostal area and finally extends into the high lobes located in the clavicular area. The air leaves the lungs in the same way, going out through the low lobes first, then the mid lobes and last the high lobes.

It is through the physical control of the three major sections of each lung that you can develop strong healthy lungs, correct any breathing difficulty and insure normal breathing patterns. Regulated, stronger lungs are especially needed in these times of impure atmospheres; our breathing habits are crucial to our lives.

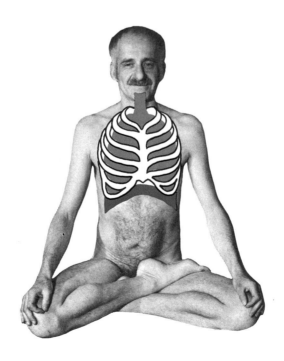

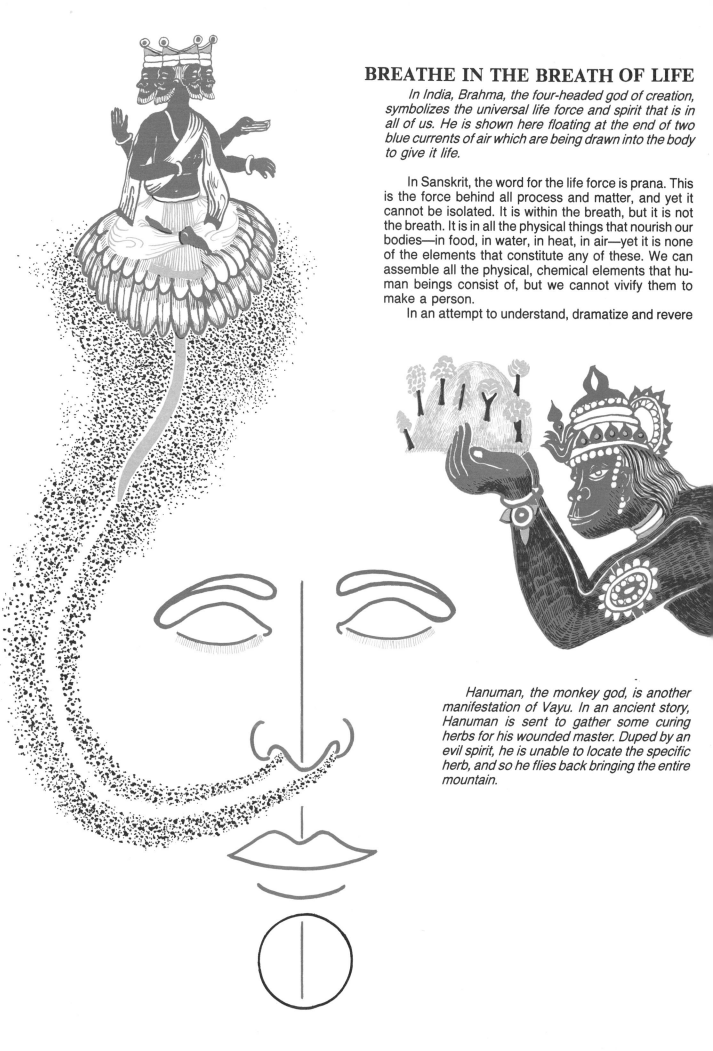

BREATHE IN THE BREATH OF LIFE

In India, Brahma, the four-headed god of creation, symbolizes the universal life force and spirit that is in all of us. He is shown here floating at the end of two blue currents of air which are being drawn into the body to give it life.

In Sanskrit, the word for the life force is prana. This is the force behind all process and matter, and yet it cannot be isolated. It is within the breath, but it is not the breath. It is in all the physical things that nourish our bodies—in food, in water, in heat, in air—yet it is none of the elements that constitute any of these. We can assemble all the physical, chemical elements that human beings consist of, but we cannot vivify them to make a person.

In an attempt to understand, dramatize and revere

Hanuman, the monkey god, is another manifestation of Vayu. In an ancient story, Hanuman is sent to gather some curing herbs for his wounded master. Duped by an evil spirit, he is unable to locate the specific herb, and so he flies back bringing the entire mountain.

this mysterious universal life force, our searching imagination has created forms in gods, concepts and symbols. As they evolve, they become interwoven in amazingly complex theological systems. Once created, these constructs can have the same life and reality as the so called material forces in our lives because they have been invested with this prana, and they have the force to influence, inspire and teach us. The most obvious manifestation of this prana is the breath within the lungs. Pranayama, one of the paths of yoga, is the science of this breath. Sectional or lobular breathing is the key to the practice of Pranayama. Through the control of our breathing, we learn how to charge the body, how to store that energy, how to still the body and mind, and how to center the mind. *Breathe in the breath of Brahma!*

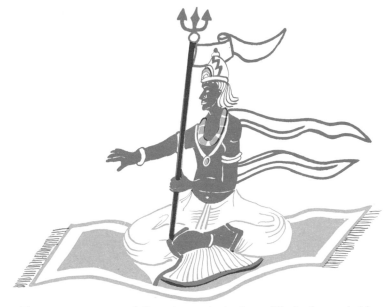

These are some of the air symbols from Hindu legend. Vayu, god and guardian of the air and wind, sails through the air.

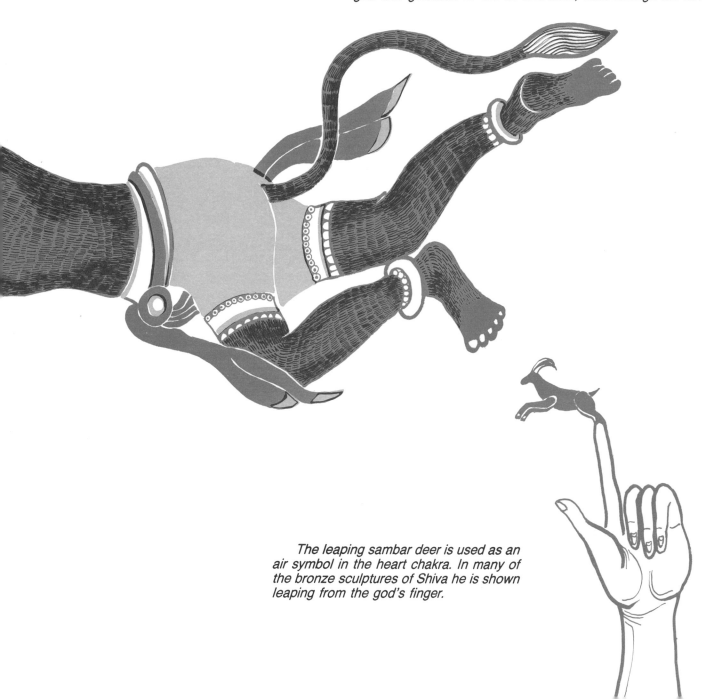

The leaping sambar deer is used as an air symbol in the heart chakra. In many of the bronze sculptures of Shiva he is shown leaping from the god's finger.

LOBULAR BREATHING ☆

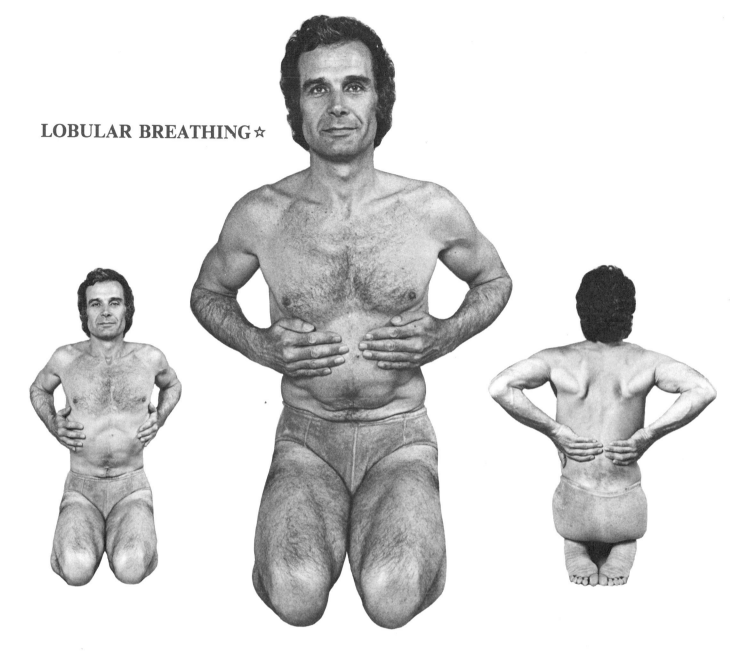

Many of our beginning students, when first taught lobular breathing, were amazed to find out what a large lung capacity they had and how little of it was actually being used.

Lower Lobe Breathing

Start to feel the depth and strength of your lungs by placing your hands on the front part of your chest in the area of the diaphragm.

Breathe deeply. As you breathe in, the lower front lobes expand, filling with air, and your hands will move outward. As you exhale, your hands come back to the original position.

After 3 to 6 rounds of this kind of breathing, move your hands to the side of your body along the outside of the lower rib cage. Breathe in deeply. Concentrate the mind into the lung area behind the hands and your hands will move outward as the lower side lobes of your lungs are filled with air. Practice this breath 3 to 6 times.

Now turn your hands around your back so that your fingers are pointing directly toward the spine. The hands are at the same level on the back of the body as the front. Through concentration on the breath, you will be able to fill this area of the lungs and thus move the hands outward.

By gaining control of the lower lobes, you will not only increase your breath and lung capacity but will tone and stimulate all of the lower organs in the abdominal and pelvic region.

Mid Lobe Breathing

Learn to open the front mid lobes of the lungs by placing one hand on the chest between the breasts. Breathe deeply in and out feeling the air fill and empty the lung area behind your hand. Do at least 3 to 6 rounds in this position.

Now place both hands along the side of the intercostal area which contains the mid lobes. Feel the rib cage move in and out as you breathe deeply in this area for 3 to 6 rounds.

Test the back mid lobes by placing the hands as far around the back mid area as possible while pointing the fingers toward the spine. Concentrate behind the hands and breathe deeply for 3 to 6 rounds.

19

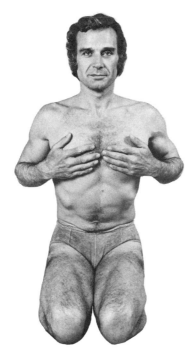
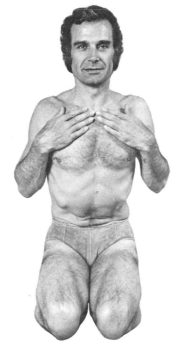

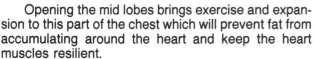

Opening the mid lobes brings exercise and expansion to this part of the chest which will prevent fat from accumulating around the heart and keep the heart muscles resilient.

Upper Lobe Breathing

The upper lobes of the lungs are the most often neglected and so contain most of the locked, residual air in the lungs. More emphasis should be placed on the exhalation in this area than the inhalation.

Bring the hands to the upper chest area just under the collar bone. Relax your shoulders and let the breath alone move your hands in and out. Great concentration is needed to fill this lung area. Do 3 to 6 rounds of this kind of breathing.

To gain control of the upper side lobes, place the hands on the hips so the lobes are free to move in and out. Now, by concentration of the mind, try to bring air in and out of the high side lobes for 3 to 6 rounds.

The upper lobes in the back are felt by raising the arms over the shoulders and placing the palms of the hands onto the back high area of the lungs. Breathe deeply and concentrate for 3 to 6 rounds. Opening the high lobes is especially helpful for anyone suffering from asthma or allergies.

You will find it beneficial to have someone work with you when first learning lobular breathing. Go through the entire routine with your partner so that he can check all of the areas of the lungs to make sure that air is flowing in and out of all of the lobes.

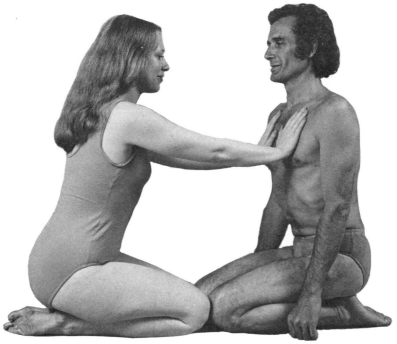

After having learned to open the lobes of your lungs, you are ready to take the deepest breath you have ever taken! On these next eight pages are a group of postures designed to expand, enlarge and rejuvenate the lobes of your lungs.

20

POSTURES TO OPEN THE LUNGS

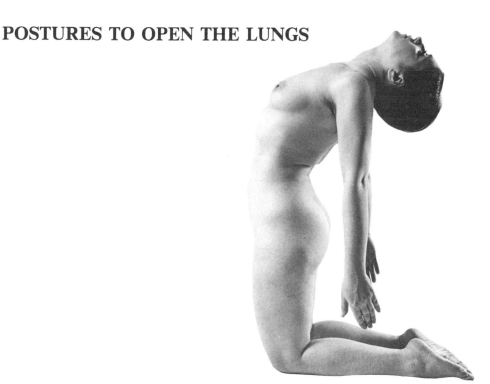

☆ The Incomplete Camel *Ustrasana*

To start opening the lower abdominal lobes of the lungs, begin with the Incomplete Camel posture. Sit on the heels in the Thunderbolt posture; exhale. On the next in-coming breath, lift the buttocks off the heels, come up onto the knees and back bend. Let the hands dangle by the sides and keep your eyes open. Sit down on the heels as you expel the breath.

The Extended Camel

In the heel sitting position, place the palms of the hands, fingers pointing up toward the top of the heel, against the soles of your feet. Pressure the hands against the feet to raise the back into a full arch, head leaning backward. Relax back to the heels. Do this posture 3 times.

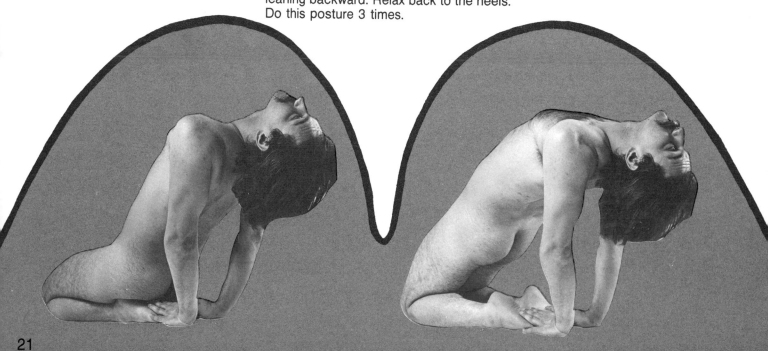

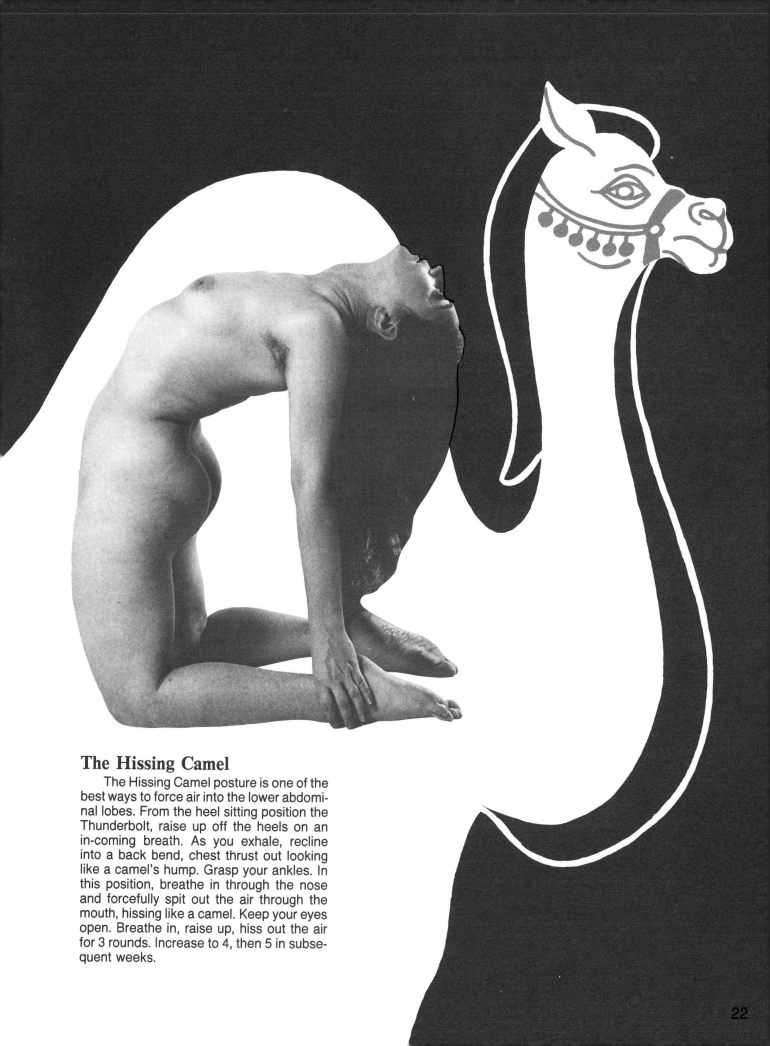

The Hissing Camel

The Hissing Camel posture is one of the best ways to force air into the lower abdominal lobes. From the heel sitting position the Thunderbolt, raise up off the heels on an in-coming breath. As you exhale, recline into a back bend, chest thrust out looking like a camel's hump. Grasp your ankles. In this position, breathe in through the nose and forcefully spit out the air through the mouth, hissing like a camel. Keep your eyes open. Breathe in, raise up, hiss out the air for 3 rounds. Increase to 4, then 5 in subsequent weeks.

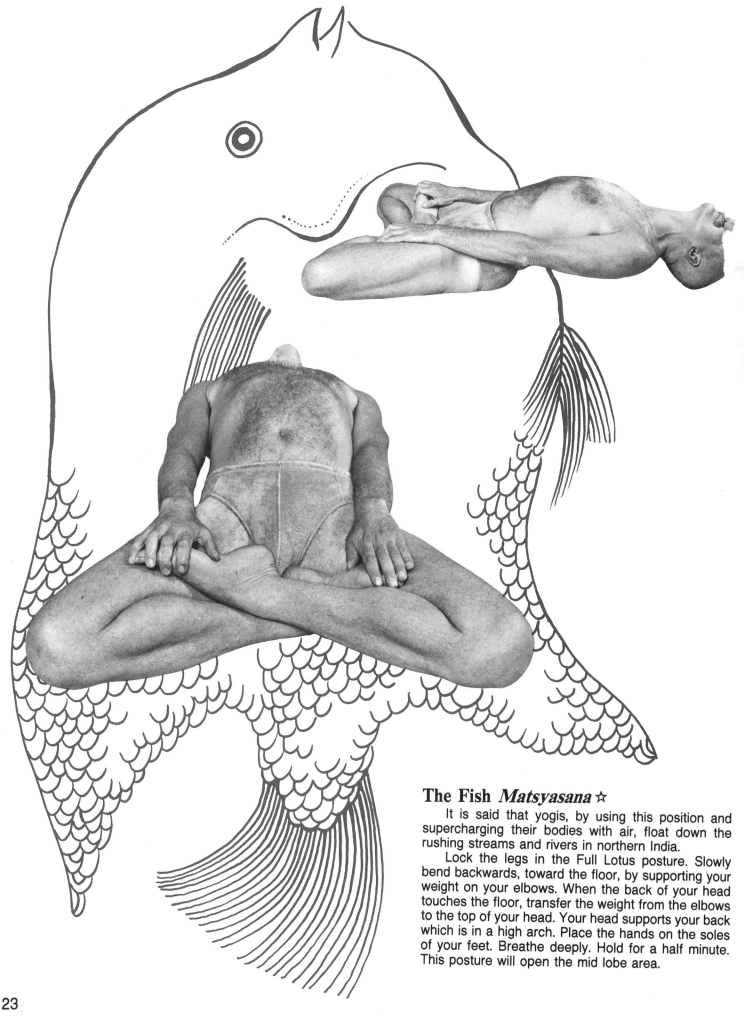

The Fish *Matsyasana* ☆

It is said that yogis, by using this position and supercharging their bodies with air, float down the rushing streams and rivers in northern India.

Lock the legs in the Full Lotus posture. Slowly bend backwards, toward the floor, by supporting your weight on your elbows. When the back of your head touches the floor, transfer the weight from the elbows to the top of your head. Your head supports your back which is in a high arch. Place the hands on the soles of your feet. Breathe deeply. Hold for a half minute. This posture will open the mid lobe area.

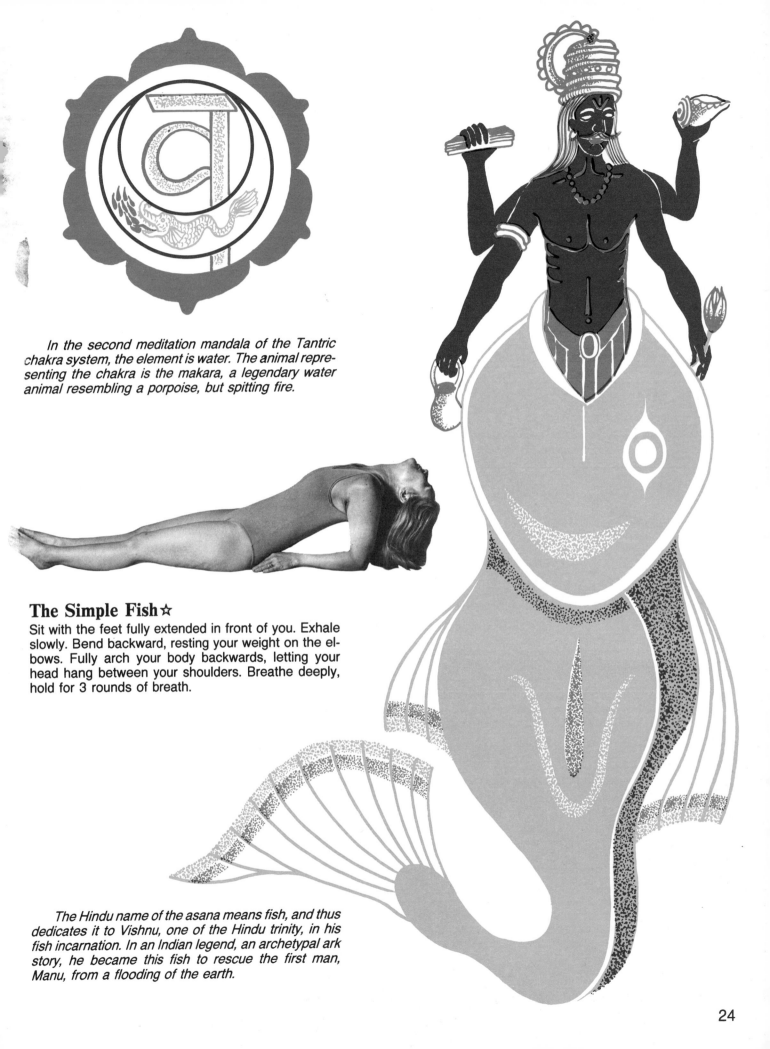

In the second meditation mandala of the Tantric chakra system, the element is water. The animal representing the chakra is the makara, a legendary water animal resembling a porpoise, but spitting fire.

The Simple Fish☆

Sit with the feet fully extended in front of you. Exhale slowly. Bend backward, resting your weight on the elbows. Fully arch your body backwards, letting your head hang between your shoulders. Breathe deeply, hold for 3 rounds of breath.

The Hindu name of the asana means fish, and thus dedicates it to Vishnu, one of the Hindu trinity, in his fish incarnation. In an Indian legend, an archetypal ark story, he became this fish to rescue the first man, Manu, from a flooding of the earth.

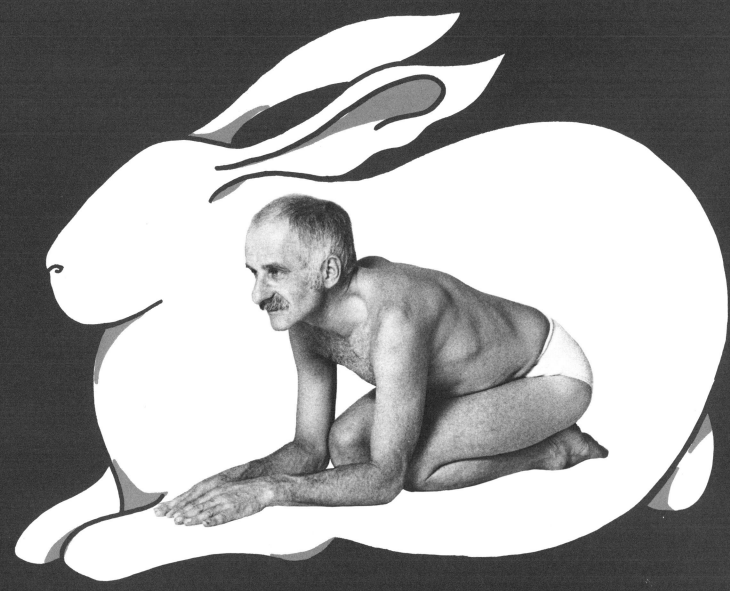

The Rabbit ☆

This Rabbit posture will open the lower and mid lobes of your lungs. You will find that as you train your lungs to expand, you will really walk with your chest thrust out, and, in turn, your posture will improve. You will become more conscious of the air around you. This can have mixed blessings in our urban situations, but in the end it is better to enlarge the lungs so that, stronger, they can better resist the scourge of air pollution. On really smoggy days breathe lightly.

Sit in the Thunderbolt posture resting on your heels. Exhale as you bend forward, resting your chest on your thighs. Your elbows are on the floor at your knees, the arms extend forward along the floor. Hold your head up high; look straight ahead. Breathe deeply in this position for 3 rounds.

The Raised Rabbit ☆

Sit in the Thunderbolt posture. Lean forward and place the palms of your hands on the floor in front of your knees. Keep your arms very straight. Hold this position, keeping the head high and pressing down on your hands. Breathe deeply for 3 rounds causing the mid lobes to expand.

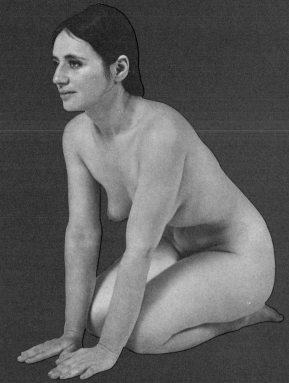

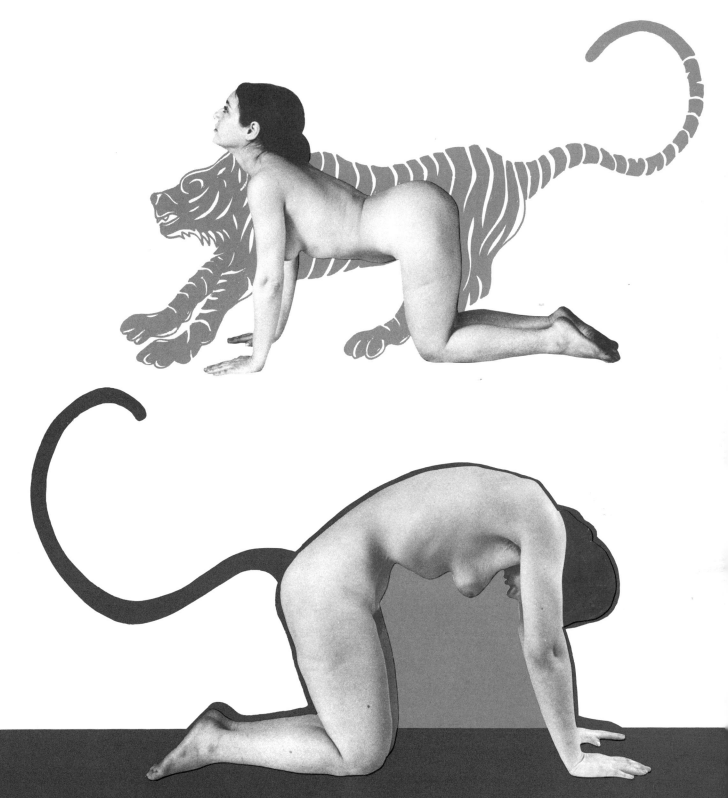

The Tiger ☆

The tiger crouches, contracting his body like a spring, preparing to leap at the exact moment.

Crouch on all fours, your body raised off the floor. Breathe in, extending the stomach downward as you slowly raise your head and neck in a taut curve.

Breathe out, bending your head down between your arms, and arch your back as high as you can.

Repeat this two-part asana 3 times. It stretches the mid lobes and is excellent for releasing tension in the spine and strengthening the nerves leading to the spinal column.

26

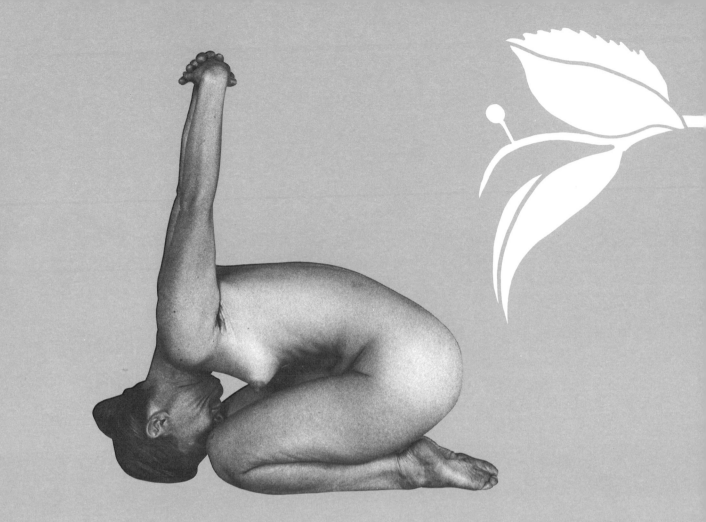

The Mighty Gesture ✧

This and the following exercise will open the high lobes of your lungs. Most people have difficulty breathing into this set of lobes, which are seldom completely filled.

Sit in the Thunderbolt posture. Clasp your hands behind your back and slowly lean forward exhaling through your mouth. The air should be completely released from your lungs by the time your upper forehead touches the floor.

Now lift your clasped hands straight up behind you. They will act as a lever to the pump that forces out most of the remaining air. Stay in this position without breath for a few seconds and then slowly sit up, taking a deep long inhalation.

Feel the air as it freshly enters your cleared lungs, first entering the low, the middle, and finally the upper lobes.

The Yoga Seal

Sit in the Lotus posture. Again clasp your hands and slowly lean forward as you exhale. Rest your chin on the floor and raise your clasped hands behind your back. Hold the posture for a few seconds with the breath held out. Then slowly lower your hands as you inhale and raise your torso to a sitting position.

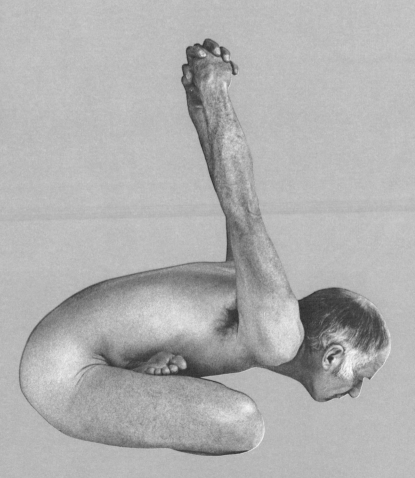

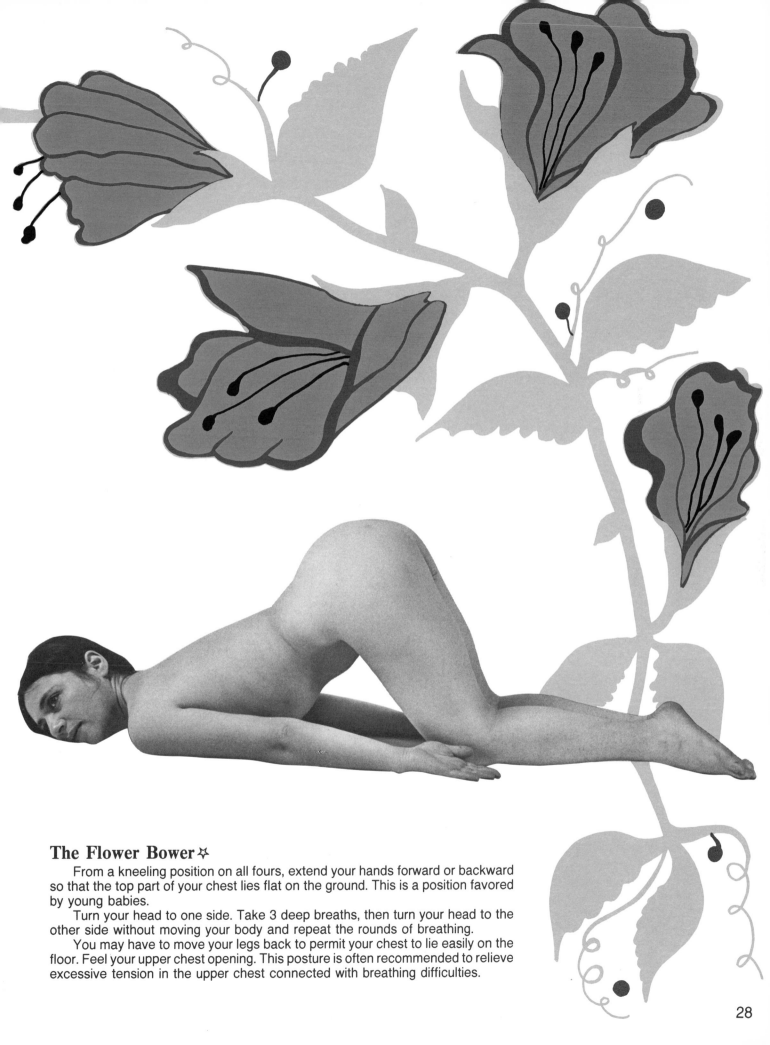

The Flower Bower ✧

From a kneeling position on all fours, extend your hands forward or backward so that the top part of your chest lies flat on the ground. This is a position favored by young babies.

Turn your head to one side. Take 3 deep breaths, then turn your head to the other side without moving your body and repeat the rounds of breathing.

You may have to move your legs back to permit your chest to lie easily on the floor. Feel your upper chest opening. This posture is often recommended to relieve excessive tension in the upper chest connected with breathing difficulties.

28

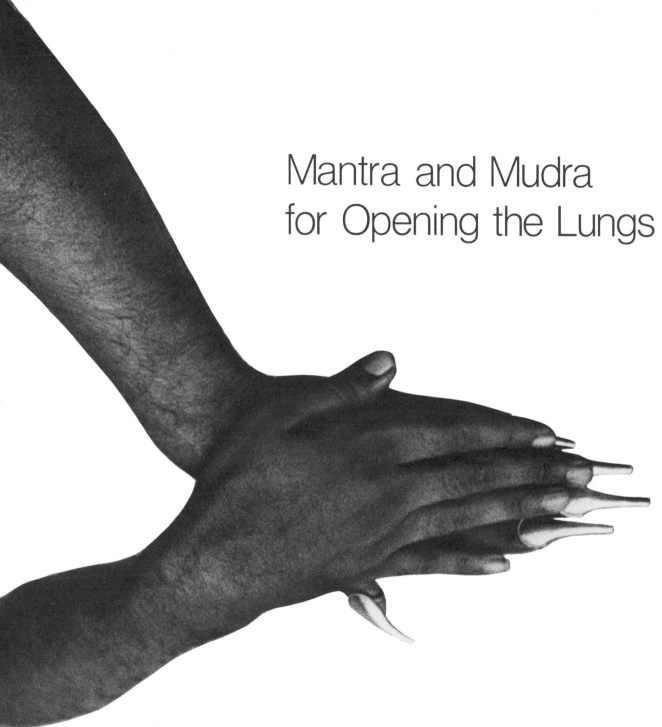

Mantra and Mudra for Opening the Lungs

The hand gestures *mudra* and sounds *mantra* connected with each section of the lungs have become part of a simple ritual which we do at the start of our yoga practice. We try to clear and expand the lungs, bring them into maximum functioning, and thereby enliven the entire body. It is a symbolic as well as a real opening up, clearing out and sychronizing for the new day.

This practice is a good introduction to mudra, the hand gestures, and to mantra, the chanting of certain vibrational sounds and words. By using mudra and mantra, you will become aware of some of the effects they have on the body in activating certain organs and nerves. The hands as well as the feet (page 12) are also nerve termi-

nals. By certain linkages of palm and fingers circuits are set up which affect the mind and body.

Mudras are also used as story-telling devices in Indian dances. The Kathakali dancer's hands, with silver talon-like extensions, mime the fish (above).

Mantra is the study in yoga and Hinduism which deals with the vibrational effect of sound. The sound of AUM which we are concentrating upon here, is thought to be the primal vibration which, when converted into its material form, created earthly-object reality.

In this exercise we use the AUM in its component parts: Ah, U, M.

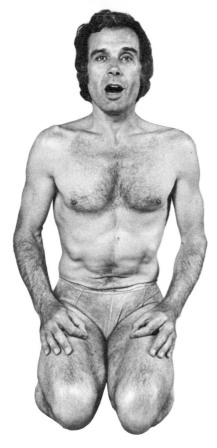

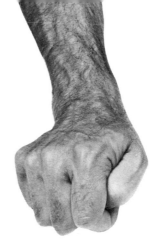
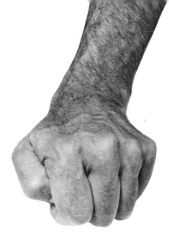

In the third gesture, curve the thumb into the palm of the hand, and fold the four fingers over it. Breathe in thinking M (mmm). Sound out the M from the high lobes as you exhale. Do this 3 times.

Make two fists, place them back to back, thumbs touching, in front of your navel. Breathe in your deepest breath as you think in the sound of Ah, U, M. Sing it out in its three distinct parts from the three sections of the lungs. Do this 3 times.

AUM Mantra ✤

Sit on your heels in the Thunderbolt posture. Put your hands on your upper thighs. Placing the hands here pressures the nerves which run to the diaphragm. The tips of the thumb and first finger are tightly touching and the other three fingers are extended close together. The fingers, by resting on the thigh, create a nerve circuit which stimulates lower lobular activity.

Breathe in deeply, slowly, thinking the sound Ah. Now sing it out as you exhale. Bring the sound from your lower lobes, a long slow extended vibrating sound. The sound Ah helps to open the lower lobes. Repeat this cycle 2 more times.

Change the hand gesture. With thumb and first finger still touching, fold under the other three fingers and press them into the palm of the hand. Breathe in thinking the sound U (ooo), exhale, sing out the U from the middle lobes. Do this 3 times.

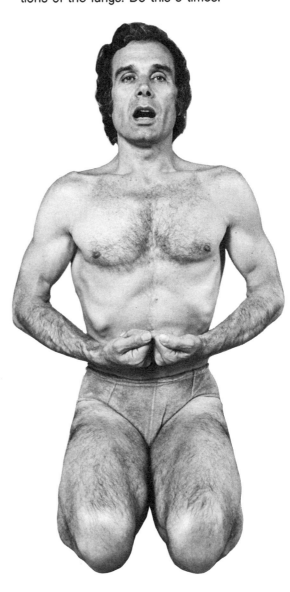

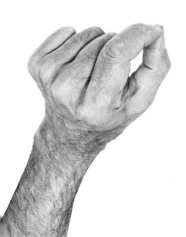
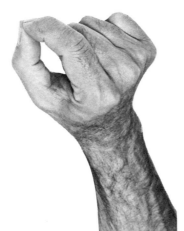

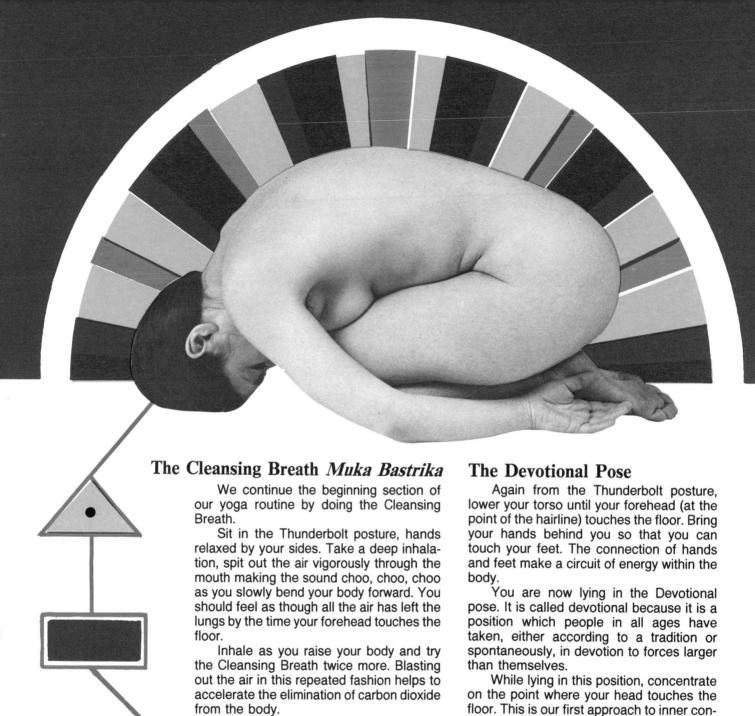

The Cleansing Breath *Muka Bastrika*

We continue the beginning section of our yoga routine by doing the Cleansing Breath.

Sit in the Thunderbolt posture, hands relaxed by your sides. Take a deep inhalation, spit out the air vigorously through the mouth making the sound choo, choo, choo as you slowly bend your body forward. You should feel as though all the air has left the lungs by the time your forehead touches the floor.

Inhale as you raise your body and try the Cleansing Breath twice more. Blasting out the air in this repeated fashion helps to accelerate the elimination of carbon dioxide from the body.

The Devotional Pose

Again from the Thunderbolt posture, lower your torso until your forehead (at the point of the hairline) touches the floor. Bring your hands behind you so that you can touch your feet. The connection of hands and feet make a circuit of energy within the body.

You are now lying in the Devotional pose. It is called devotional because it is a position which people in all ages have taken, either according to a tradition or spontaneously, in devotion to forces larger than themselves.

While lying in this position, concentrate on the point where your head touches the floor. This is our first approach to inner concentration.

At this point visualize a black dot, a wall of your favorite color, or the sun. When concentrating on the sun, as you watch it interiorly, imagine a total sunrise, from the first rays of dawn to the full sun shining in your head. Hold the position and concentration for at least a minute.

This concludes our beginning routine of opening the lungs, spitting out the breath, and concentrating the mind.

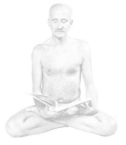
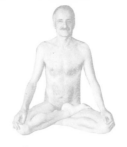

Using the Book, Using the Body

Try to do your daily practice in a quiet, neat place of moderate temperature, with fresh air but no drafts. It could be a space specially reserved for yoga with a special mat or rug. If we are ready to make a separate place in our homes for sleeping, eating, washing, and tv watching, we should do the same for yoga.

Working out-of-doors is excellent, when possible. However, nature's vibrations can sometimes be overpowering and diverting, so either surrender to them at the time or, if you are really intent on the practice, pursue the yoga and the concentration will come. Then nature can serve as a reinforcing background.

As you do the yoga, abandon yourself to the rhythmic feelings in your body. Watching your own body's movements will bring you into a new awareness of the unbelievably complex and miraculous apparatus that the body is.

Watching the body movements leads you into a mood of awareness which makes yoga transcend ordinary exercise—to become an exercise of the spirit. Done in this contained spirit, confining your attention to the posture you are doing will increase your power of concentration. You will find that ordinary consciousness falls away and you will be practicing on a plane of consciousness much higher than the one you usually live on. Time consciousness will also fall away.

One of our teachers would always ask, after each asana, if we had any outside thoughts, testing us to see how really concentrated and contained we were.

The next few pages will show you how to coordinate the breath with the asanas. There follows a selection of almost one hundred postures from the thousands of postures in yoga.

The order in which you learn the postures can vary. It is best to start with postures that will come to you most easily. The easiest postures, for beginners, are indicated by a star (*) next to the name of the asana, and it is suggested that you try these first. This is not a strict rule as different bodies sometimes will find different postures easier.

The easy postures will open the body, release tension and enable you to do more complicated poses. Using this method of easy postures leading into more difficult ones, you will slowly build a rigorous daily practice.

You should always do your yoga on a soft but firm surface, to buffer the body against the hard floor or ground.

An effort has been made to have each page of postures flow into the next. This is the spirit in which you should coordinate the postures you choose to do each day.

Your practice should combine lying, sitting and standing poses and some of the classic postures and should conclude with the breathing exercises. Give emphasis to parts of the body that need special attention.

Try to do a routine that will fit into your daily life. Ten minutes will be beneficial, a half hour is very good, an hour is ideal. Establish a rhythm by trying not to miss a day. If, as in many of our lives, you are forced to give up the practice for a time, start up again slowly, patiently, with the simple asanas.

If you can occasionally do your asanas in front of a large mirror, it will help you to refine the postures.

Do not strain in a posture. Each time you do the asana your body will tend to be more flexible in it. But the benefits of the yoga will not show immediately. The rebuilding of the body can only take place slowly. Yoga cannot always change the chronic body difficulties of the new student, but it usually will arrest them and prevent many new troubles from starting.

In most of the sitting and lying postures, where balance is not critical, we do yoga with our eyes closed. It deepens the concentration. Each posture is usually done three times, on either side, to the Rhythmic Breath. The instructions will specifically state this in the following few exercises, but it will be taken for granted later on, unless other directions are given.

Teachers have different styles and paces, resulting from their own experience of the rich field of yoga. Many work with groups; some believe the way is through individual instruction.

We knew one teacher who held each student in a most loving manner as he worked with them, combining a kind of chiropractic adjustment with the yoga to loosen their bodies for the asanas.

Some stress that the posture should be done three times, others that the asana be done only once. Actually these are two stages of progress. The repeated rhythm of a single asana that we stress in this book opens the body. The very advanced student, having fully opened the body, can then get the posture's full effect by doing it just once.

Some teach that you should feel pain when doing an asana, that pain is a sign of the body changing. This can be a dangerous point of view, especially without very careful supervision.

In India, we used to hear the term "Bogha Yoga" used in a pejorative sense. We thought at first that "Bogha" had something to do with bogus and, in a roundabout way, it did; for "Bogha" is the Hindi word for enjoyment and thus "Bogha Yoga" meant nonserious yoga. One *should* do yoga with the spirit of present joy, however. To do it only for austerity, for body building, or as preparation for other disciplines robs it of one of its essential aspects.

One of our teachers would loudly ask, after we had done an asana, "Did you get satisfaction?" Did you feel the full enjoyment of doing the posture?

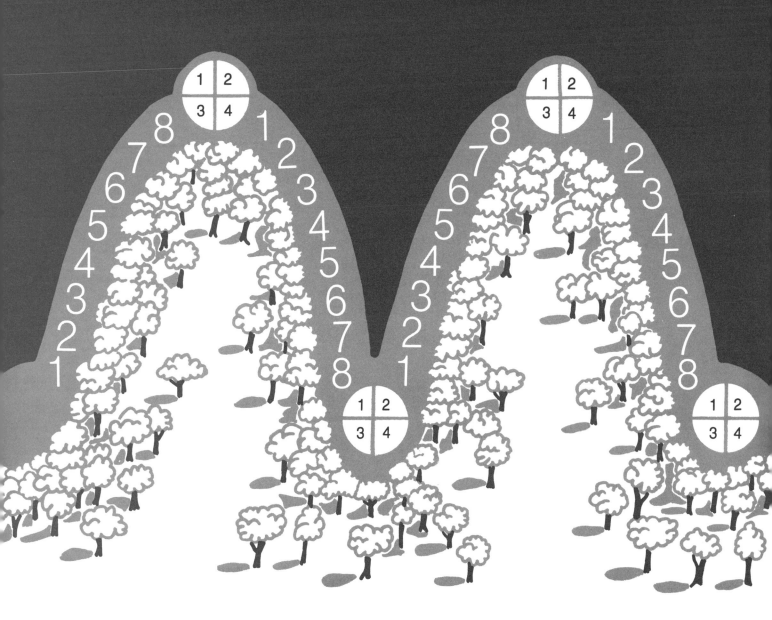

THE RHYTHMIC BREATH SAVITRI PRANAYAMA

Inhale	Hold in	Exhale	Hold out	
8	4	8	4	for the physical body
6	3	6	3	for the emotional body

Sit in any relaxed sitting position with a straight back. Breathe in and out slowly. Now draw in the breath for the count of 6, hold for the count of 3, exhale for the count of 6, and hold out the breath for the count of 3. Do this for 6 rounds. Now try to increase the ratio so that the breathing pattern is 8–4–8–4. Do this for 6 rounds.

In this breathing cycle you pull in the prana, the life energy, retain it so it can be absorbed, and then expel the wastes. When all the air is expelled, you permit the body to be at rest. By this process you also train the body to increase its consumption of air.

These breath patterns are named after the beauti-

ful goddess Savitri who, in one of the classic Hindu tales, challenges the god of death, Yama, and convinces him to abandon his designs on her husband's life. And so, giver of life is Savitri, and giver of life is this Savitri breath.

This pattern should be used in other physical movements in your life like walking, lifting and climbing. It makes for even, controlled, unstrained motion.

The 6–3–6–3 rhythm of breath affects the emotions and should be used whenever one feels emotionally distraught. Pausing to do this simple breathing pattern will help to calm and relax you.

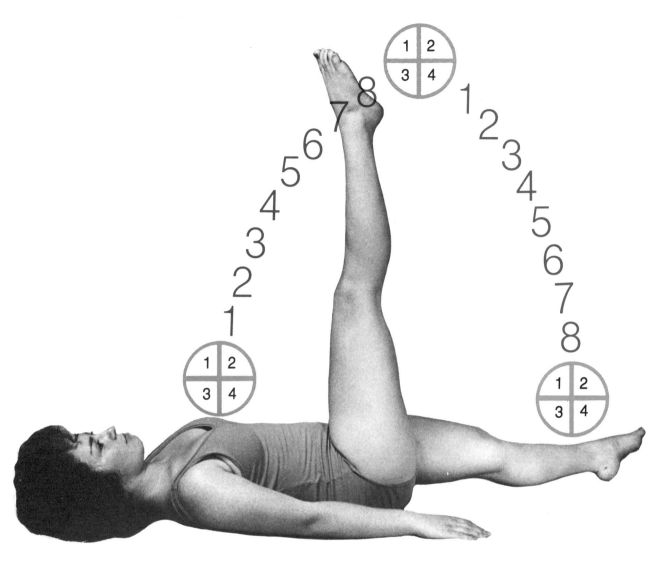

Single and Double Leg Lift to the Breath ✡

Lie on the floor. Do a few rounds of the 6–3–6–3 breath. Slowly lift your right leg, knee straight, for the count of 6 on the in-breath. Keep your leg in the air while holding the breath for the count of 3. Slowly, lower your leg to the floor for the count of 6 as you let out the breath. Lie still with the breath suspended for the count of 3. Do this 3 times on either side. Now, raise both legs to the same rhythm, for 3 rounds.

You have now coordinated the rhythmic yoga breath with this yoga posture. This kind of breath pattern will be used with most of the postures.

After a few days, when you have accustomed your body to the 6–3–6–3 rhythm, change to the 8–4–8–4, which will be the one you will use permanently for all of your exercises. After awhile, breath rhythm and body rhythm will become so well paced and integrated that you will no longer need to count.

Having done the front leg lifts, we now do a set of lifting positions which move around the body, beginning with the side.

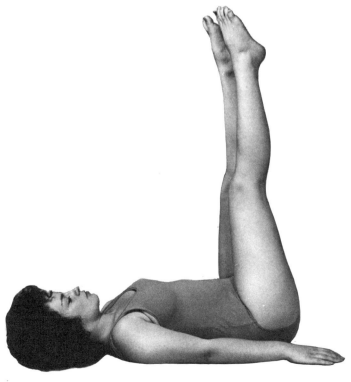

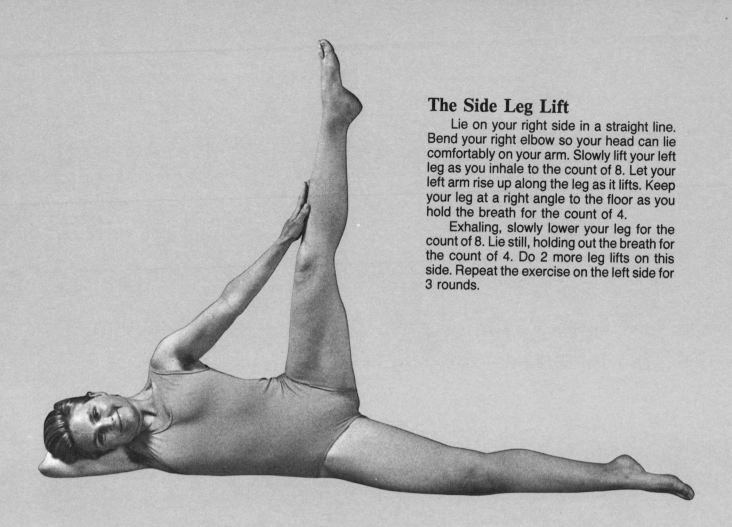

The Side Leg Lift

Lie on your right side in a straight line. Bend your right elbow so your head can lie comfortably on your arm. Slowly lift your left leg as you inhale to the count of 8. Let your left arm rise up along the leg as it lifts. Keep your leg at a right angle to the floor as you hold the breath for the count of 4.

Exhaling, slowly lower your leg for the count of 8. Lie still, holding out the breath for the count of 4. Do 2 more leg lifts on this side. Repeat the exercise on the left side for 3 rounds.

The Double Side Leg Lift

Lie on your right side in the same position as the Side Leg Lift. Place your left hand in front of your body at waist level. The palm of your hand pressures the floor as you lift your legs. Using the Rhythmic Breath, slowly lift both legs, hold, lower and rest.

Repeat 2 more times and then do it on the left side. This posture will be more difficult at first than the single leg lift; daily practice will help you to attain your highest lift.

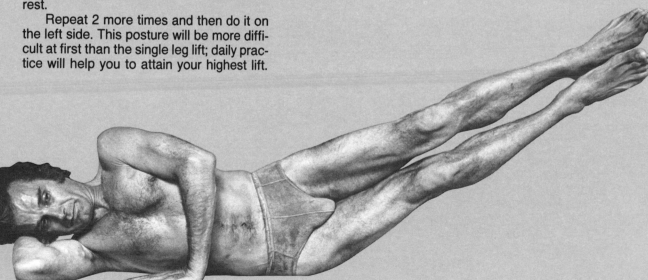

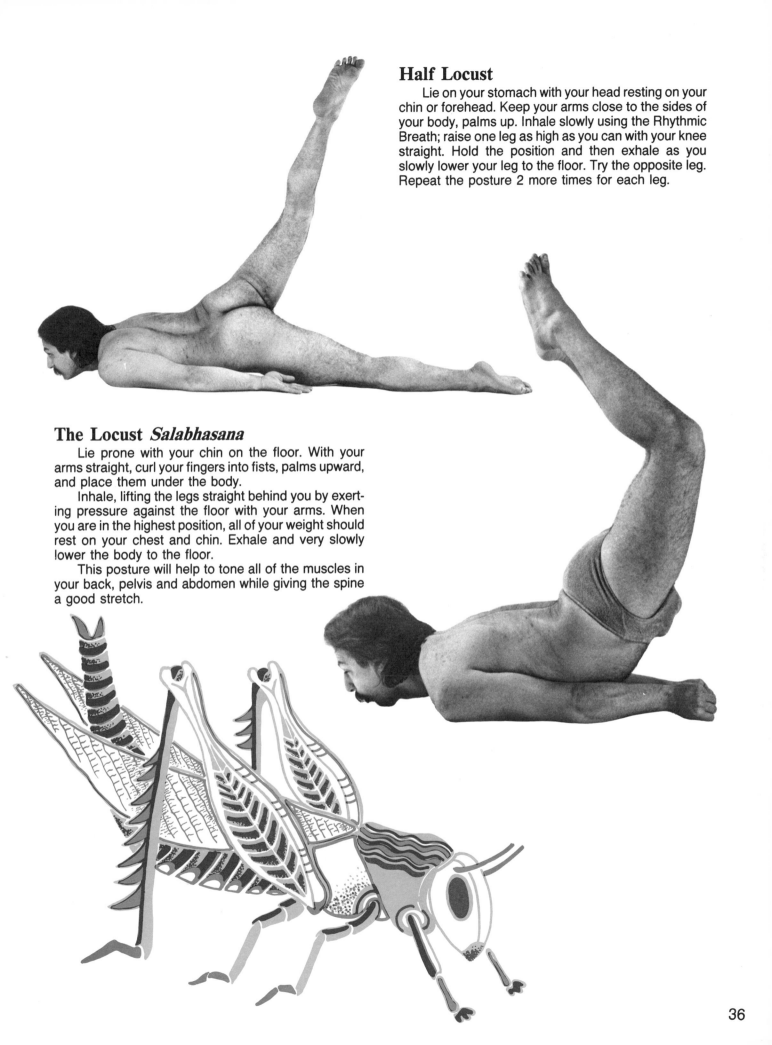

Half Locust

Lie on your stomach with your head resting on your chin or forehead. Keep your arms close to the sides of your body, palms up. Inhale slowly using the Rhythmic Breath; raise one leg as high as you can with your knee straight. Hold the position and then exhale as you slowly lower your leg to the floor. Try the opposite leg. Repeat the posture 2 more times for each leg.

The Locust *Salabhasana*

Lie prone with your chin on the floor. With your arms straight, curl your fingers into fists, palms upward, and place them under the body.

Inhale, lifting the legs straight behind you by exerting pressure against the floor with your arms. When you are in the highest position, all of your weight should rest on your chest and chin. Exhale and very slowly lower the body to the floor.

This posture will help to tone all of the muscles in your back, pelvis and abdomen while giving the spine a good stretch.

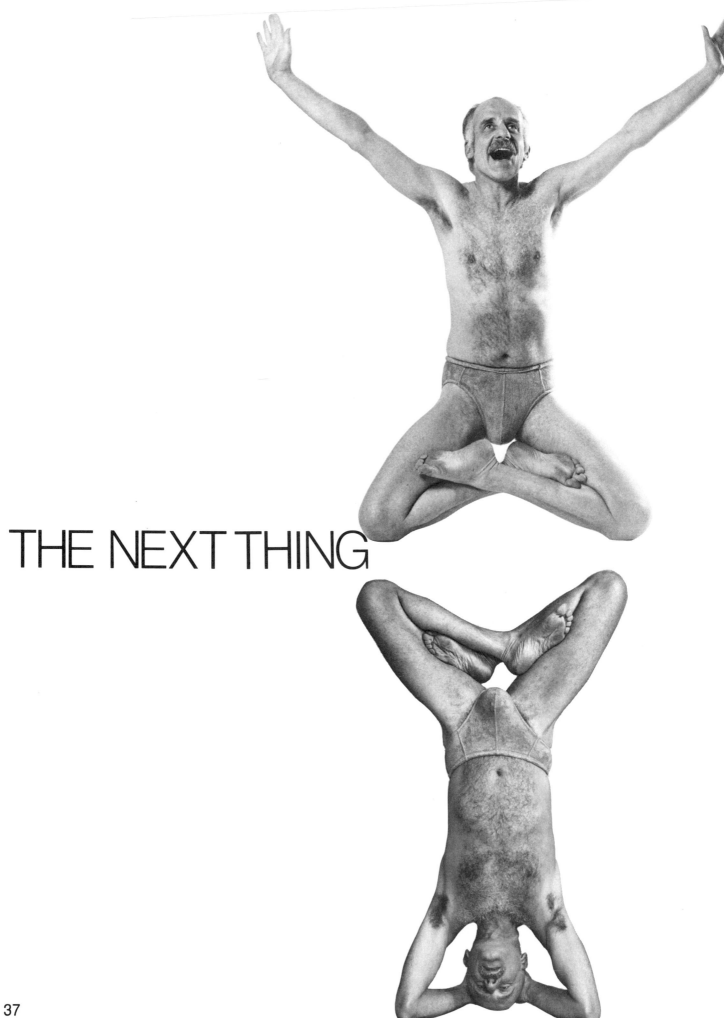

THE NEXT THING

YOU MUST LEARN IS A SERIES
OF ASANAS

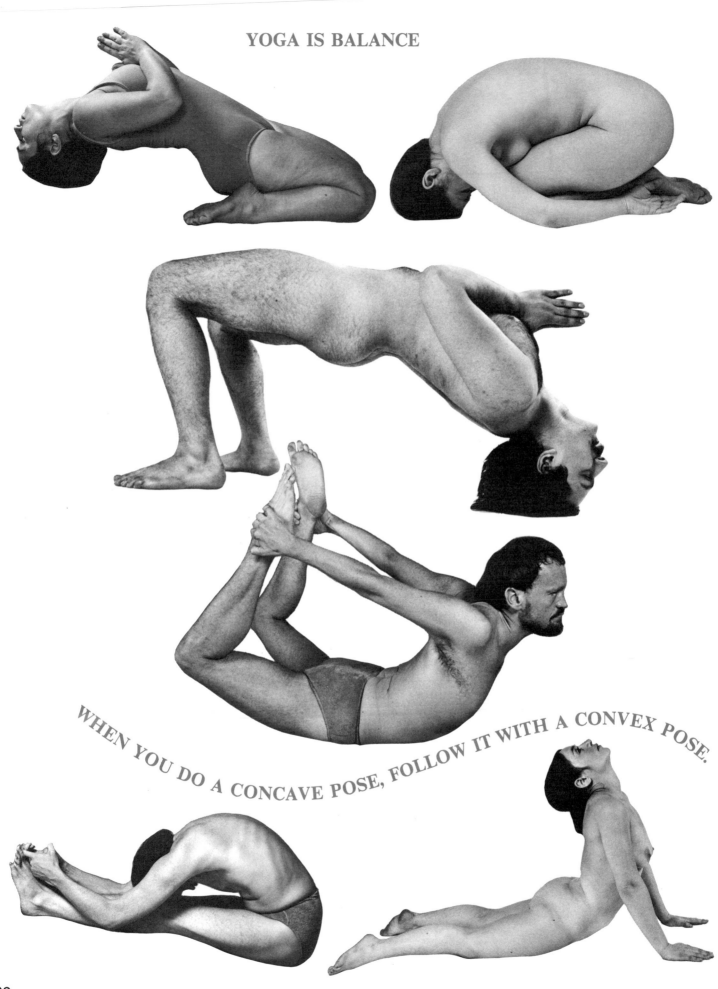

YOGA IS BALANCE

WHEN YOU DO A CONCAVE POSE, FOLLOW IT WITH A CONVEX POSE.

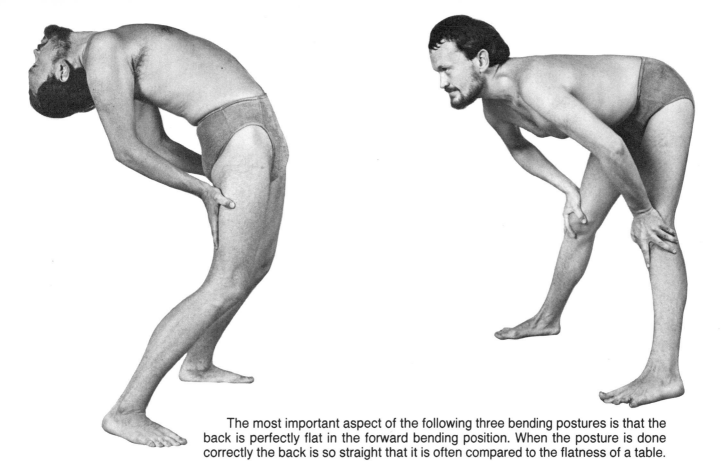

The most important aspect of the following three bending postures is that the back is perfectly flat in the forward bending position. When the posture is done correctly the back is so straight that it is often compared to the flatness of a table.

Bend to the Knees ☆

Stand with your legs spread an arm and a half's length apart. Point your feet straight ahead. Use the Rhythmic Breath. On the out-breath, bend forward from the lower back until you feel your torso is in a parallel position to the floor. Hold this position with your hands on top of your knees. Inhale, lift into a straight standing position and hold.

Exhaling, backbend, slide your hands down along the back of your legs, using them if necessary to support your back. Keep your eyes open or you may lose your balance. Hold at the lowest point of the backbend. Inhale as you lift into a straight standing position again.

Bend to the Floor ☆

Place your hands on your hips. Now spread your legs as wide as you can and keep your feet pointing straight ahead. Slowly bend forward, this time touching your head to the floor. Do the backbend as a balance to the forward position.

This is a more difficult posture than the Bend to the Knees. The head should be as close in line with the feet as possible.

These postures will bring great flexibility to the spine.

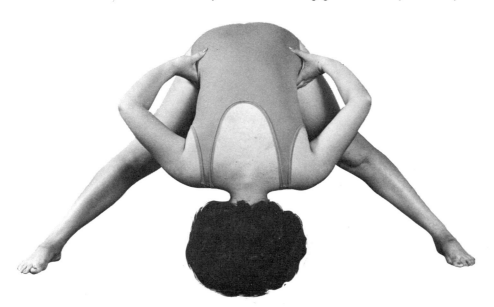

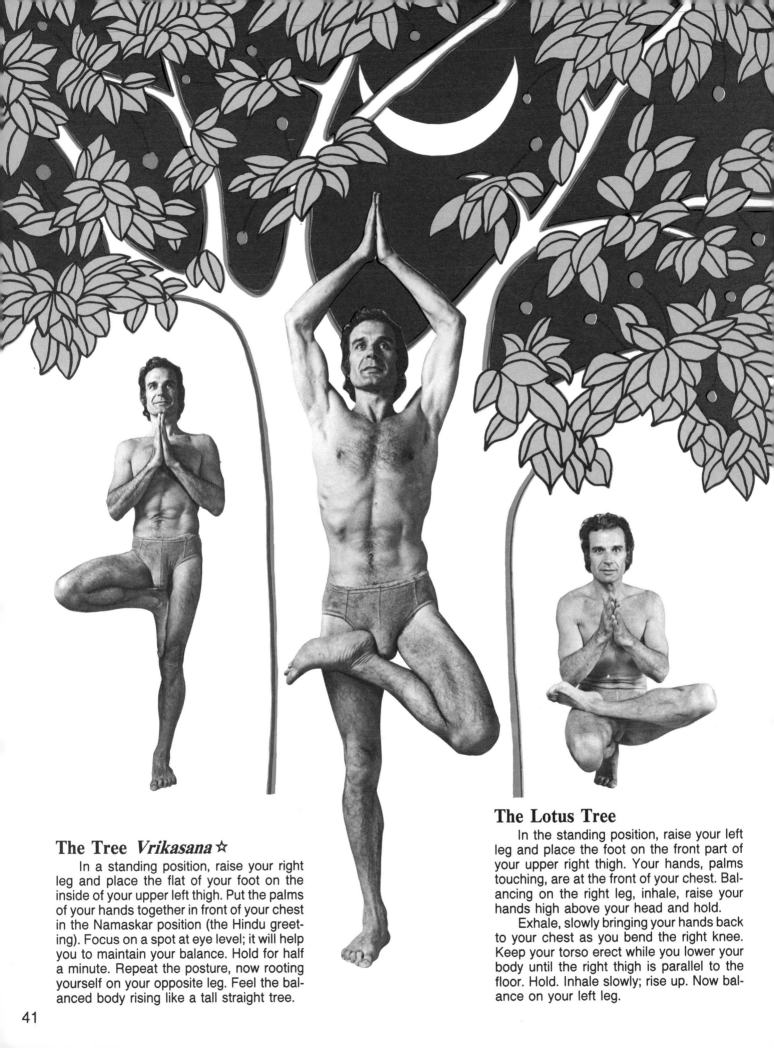

The Tree *Vrikasana* ☆

In a standing position, raise your right leg and place the flat of your foot on the inside of your upper left thigh. Put the palms of your hands together in front of your chest in the Namaskar position (the Hindu greeting). Focus on a spot at eye level; it will help you to maintain your balance. Hold for half a minute. Repeat the posture, now rooting yourself on your opposite leg. Feel the balanced body rising like a tall straight tree.

The Lotus Tree

In the standing position, raise your left leg and place the foot on the front part of your upper right thigh. Your hands, palms touching, are at the front of your chest. Balancing on the right leg, inhale, raise your hands high above your head and hold.

Exhale, slowly bringing your hands back to your chest as you bend the right knee. Keep your torso erect while you lower your body until the right thigh is parallel to the floor. Hold. Inhale slowly; rise up. Now balance on your left leg.

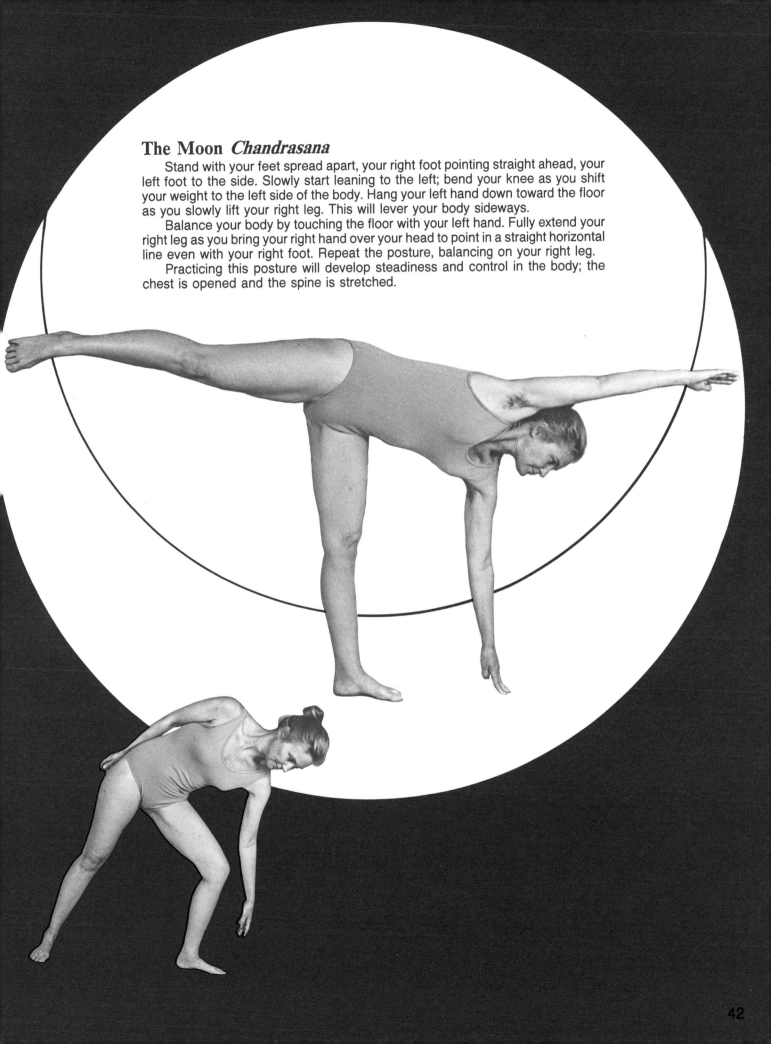

The Moon *Chandrasana*

Stand with your feet spread apart, your right foot pointing straight ahead, your left foot to the side. Slowly start leaning to the left; bend your knee as you shift your weight to the left side of the body. Hang your left hand down toward the floor as you slowly lift your right leg. This will lever your body sideways.

Balance your body by touching the floor with your left hand. Fully extend your right leg as you bring your right hand over your head to point in a straight horizontal line even with your right foot. Repeat the posture, balancing on your right leg.

Practicing this posture will develop steadiness and control in the body; the chest is opened and the spine is stretched.

Every time you do these postures, be aware of the different triangular structures formed by the body.

☆ The Basic Triangle *Trikonasana*

Stand with your feet apart about one arm's length, right foot pointing forward, left foot to the side. Inhale, lifting your arms sideways to shoulder level. Hold. Exhale while slowly bending the trunk of your body to the left side until your left hand touches your left foot. Your right hand is raised straight above you, palm forward. The head is turned so that you can look up at your hand.

Try to keep your arms, chest, hips and legs in a straight line while holding the position. Inhale and raise your body, letting your arms drop to your sides. Repeat the posture on both sides 3 times.

The Twisting Triangle

Start with the arms spread wide apart. Exhaling, bend from the waist, swinging the torso so that the left hand touches the right foot. Look up at your right hand which is extended upward. Keep your legs straight. Rise up on the in-breath.

These two exercises make the entire spinal area more supple.

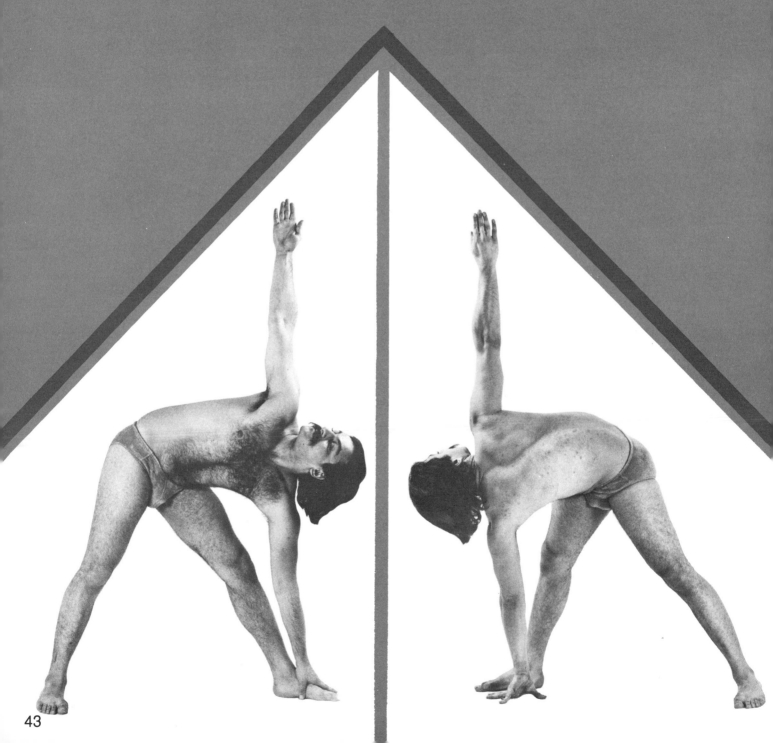

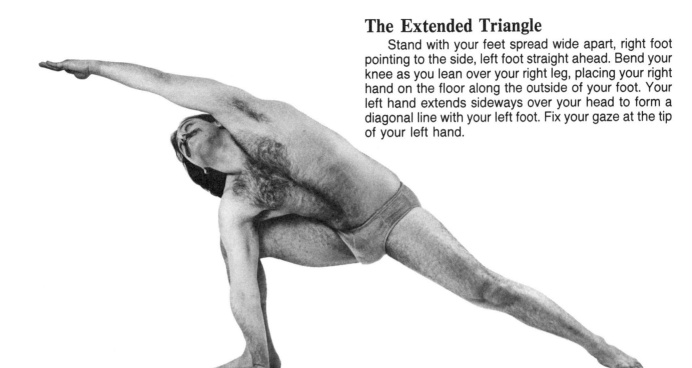

The Extended Triangle

Stand with your feet spread wide apart, right foot pointing to the side, left foot straight ahead. Bend your knee as you lean over your right leg, placing your right hand on the floor along the outside of your foot. Your left hand extends sideways over your head to form a diagonal line with your left foot. Fix your gaze at the tip of your left hand.

The Poised Arrow *Virabhadrasana*

Stand with your feet one arm's length apart. Point your left foot toward the side, horizontally in line with your right heel. Place your hands in front of your chest, palms touching. Inhale as you raise your hands straight above your head and then hold. Exhale as you lower your hands back to the front of your chest.

On the next in-breath, twist your body to the left side. Exhale while stretching your arms and torso forward over your left leg and slowly lift your right leg straight up behind you. From hand to heel the body should be in a straight line parallel to the floor. Reverse the steps and return to the first position. Repeat this posture 3 times on each side.

In this asana the body learns balance by a cantilevered stretch in either direction.

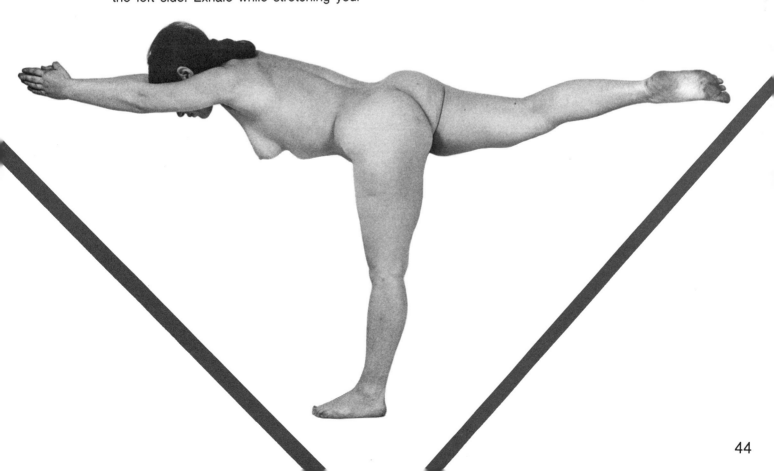

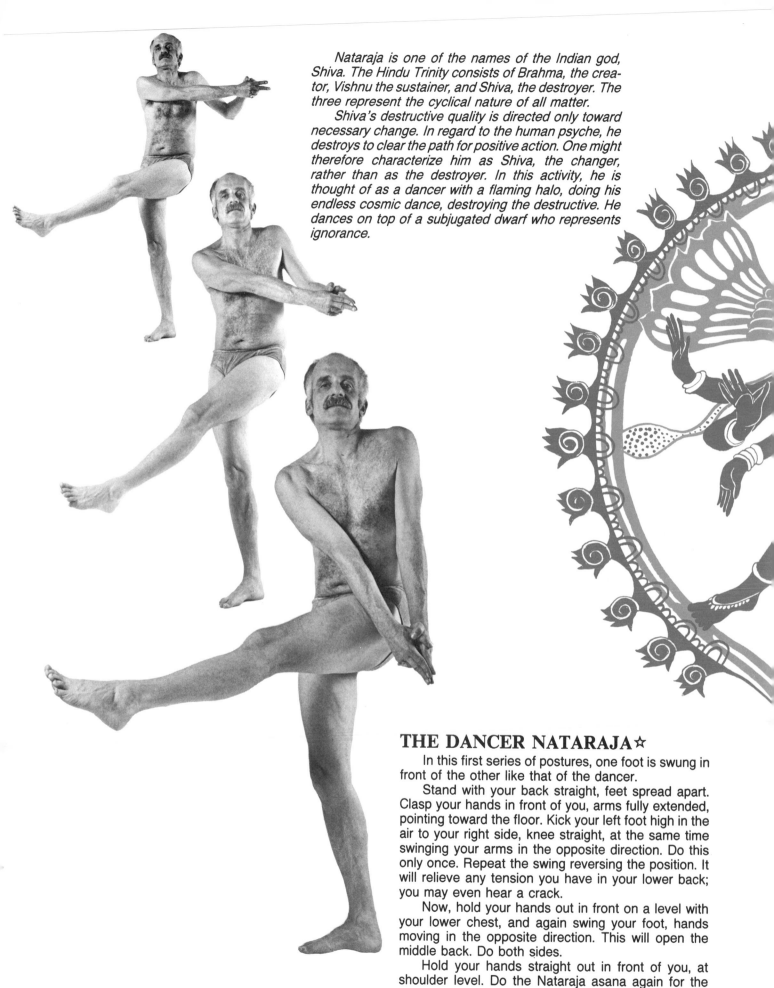

Nataraja is one of the names of the Indian god, Shiva. The Hindu Trinity consists of Brahma, the creator, Vishnu the sustainer, and Shiva, the destroyer. The three represent the cyclical nature of all matter.

Shiva's destructive quality is directed only toward necessary change. In regard to the human psyche, he destroys to clear the path for positive action. One might therefore characterize him as Shiva, the changer, rather than as the destroyer. In this activity, he is thought of as a dancer with a flaming halo, doing his endless cosmic dance, destroying the destructive. He dances on top of a subjugated dwarf who represents ignorance.

THE DANCER NATARAJA ☆

In this first series of postures, one foot is swung in front of the other like that of the dancer.

Stand with your back straight, feet spread apart. Clasp your hands in front of you, arms fully extended, pointing toward the floor. Kick your left foot high in the air to your right side, knee straight, at the same time swinging your arms in the opposite direction. Do this only once. Repeat the swing reversing the position. It will relieve any tension you have in your lower back; you may even hear a crack.

Now, hold your hands out in front on a level with your lower chest, and again swing your foot, hands moving in the opposite direction. This will open the middle back. Do both sides.

Hold your hands straight out in front of you, at shoulder level. Do the Nataraja asana again for the upper part of your back.

45

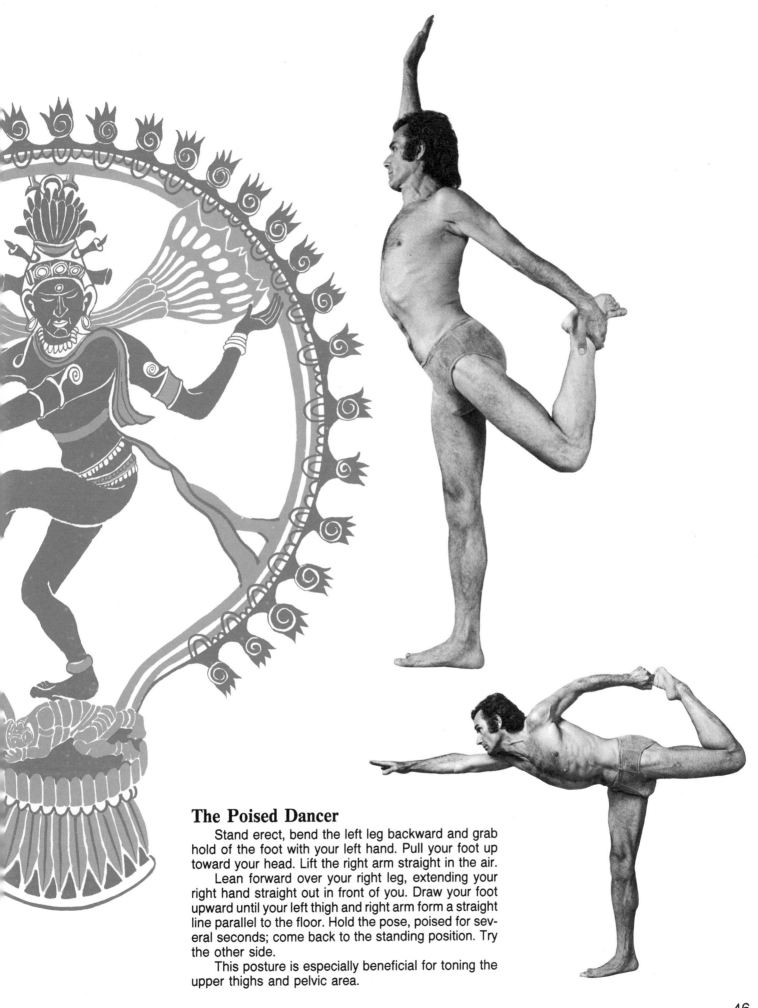

The Poised Dancer

Stand erect, bend the left leg backward and grab hold of the foot with your left hand. Pull your foot up toward your head. Lift the right arm straight in the air.

Lean forward over your right leg, extending your right hand straight out in front of you. Draw your foot upward until your left thigh and right arm form a straight line parallel to the floor. Hold the pose, poised for several seconds; come back to the standing position. Try the other side.

This posture is especially beneficial for toning the upper thighs and pelvic area.

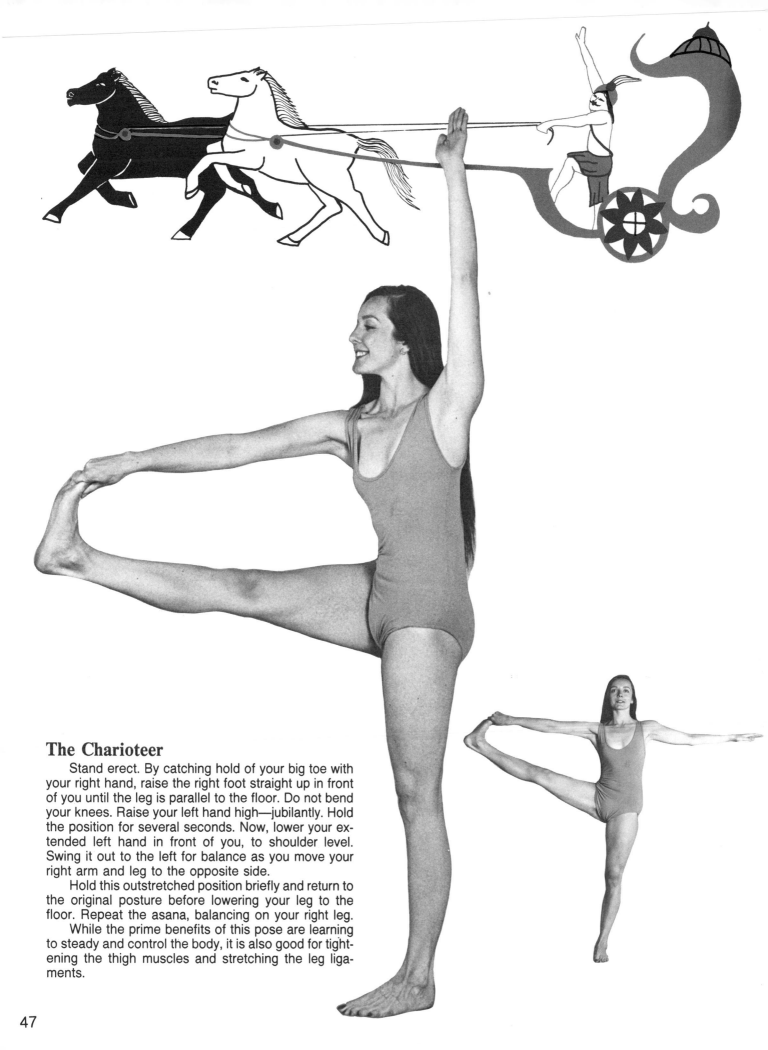

The Charioteer

Stand erect. By catching hold of your big toe with your right hand, raise the right foot straight up in front of you until the leg is parallel to the floor. Do not bend your knees. Raise your left hand high—jubilantly. Hold the position for several seconds. Now, lower your extended left hand in front of you, to shoulder level. Swing it out to the left for balance as you move your right arm and leg to the opposite side.

Hold this outstretched position briefly and return to the original posture before lowering your leg to the floor. Repeat the asana, balancing on your right leg.

While the prime benefits of this pose are learning to steady and control the body, it is also good for tightening the thigh muscles and stretching the leg ligaments.

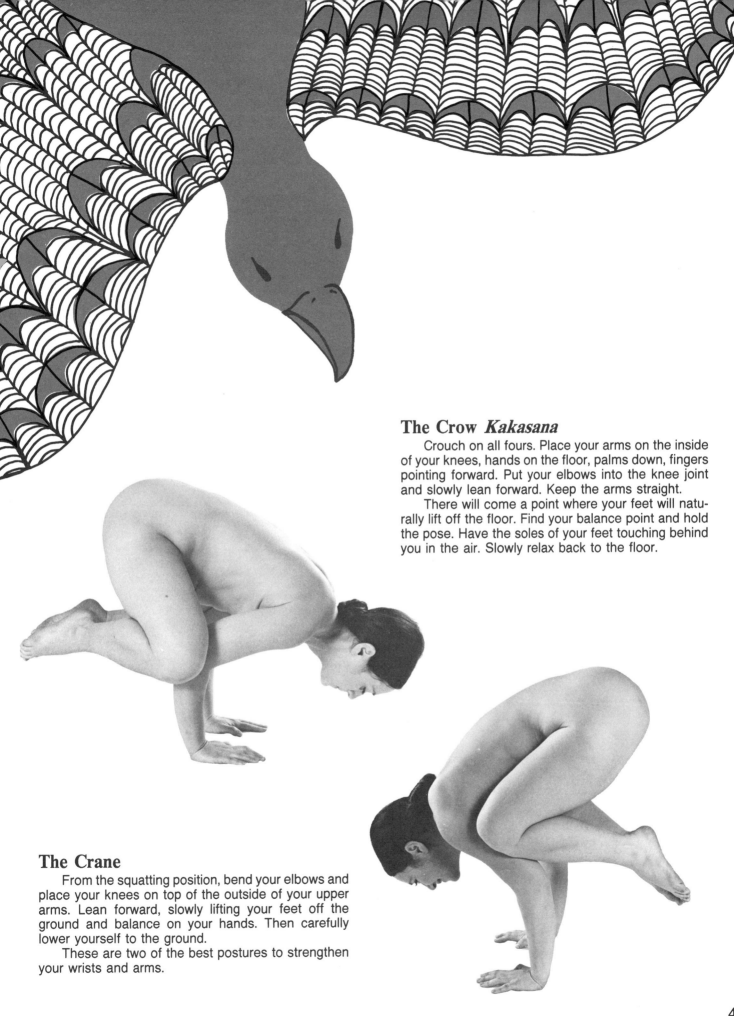

The Crow *Kakasana*

Crouch on all fours. Place your arms on the inside of your knees, hands on the floor, palms down, fingers pointing forward. Put your elbows into the knee joint and slowly lean forward. Keep the arms straight.

There will come a point where your feet will naturally lift off the floor. Find your balance point and hold the pose. Have the soles of your feet touching behind you in the air. Slowly relax back to the floor.

The Crane

From the squatting position, bend your elbows and place your knees on top of the outside of your upper arms. Lean forward, slowly lifting your feet off the ground and balance on your hands. Then carefully lower yourself to the ground.

These are two of the best postures to strengthen your wrists and arms.

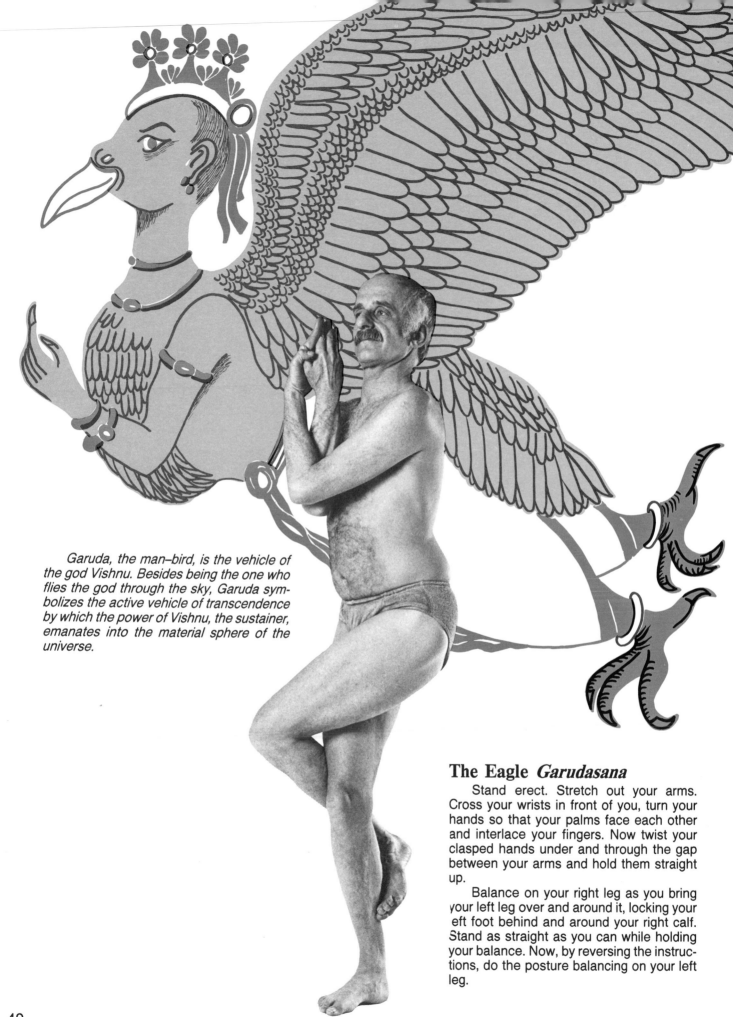

Garuda, the man–bird, is the vehicle of the god Vishnu. Besides being the one who flies the god through the sky, Garuda symbolizes the active vehicle of transcendence by which the power of Vishnu, the sustainer, emanates into the material sphere of the universe.

The Eagle *Garudasana*

Stand erect. Stretch out your arms. Cross your wrists in front of you, turn your hands so that your palms face each other and interlace your fingers. Now twist your clasped hands under and through the gap between your arms and hold them straight up.

Balance on your right leg as you bring your left leg over and around it, locking your left foot behind and around your right calf. Stand as straight as you can while holding your balance. Now, by reversing the instructions, do the posture balancing on your left leg.

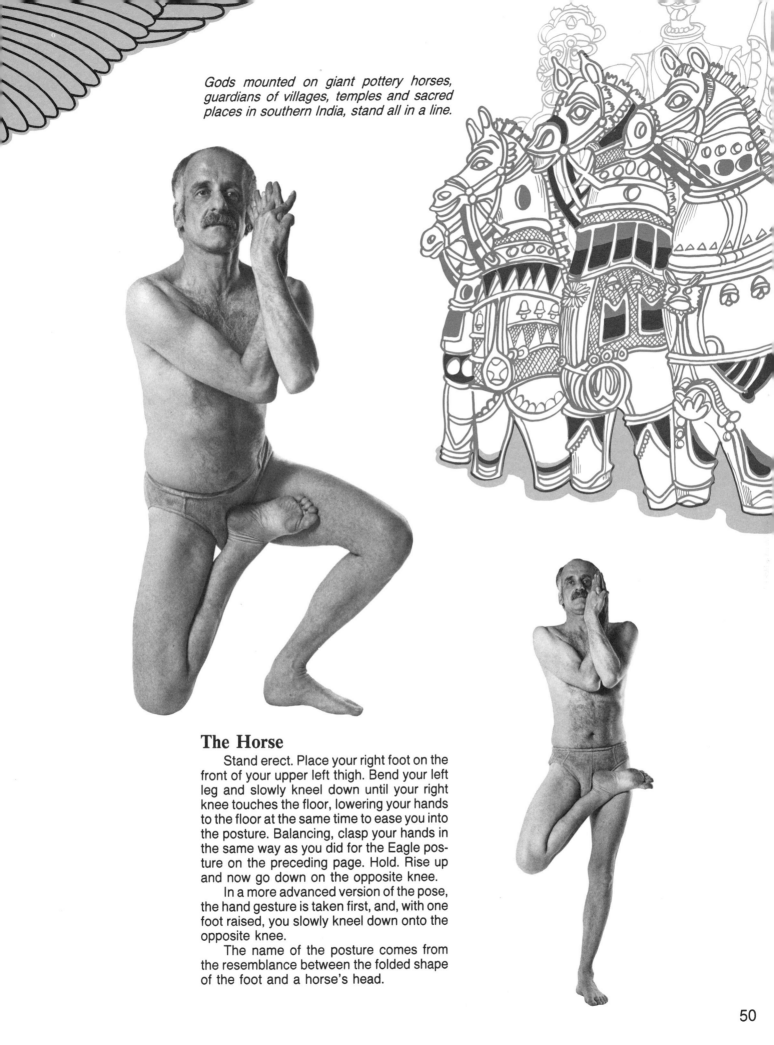

Gods mounted on giant pottery horses, guardians of villages, temples and sacred places in southern India, stand all in a line.

The Horse

Stand erect. Place your right foot on the front of your upper left thigh. Bend your left leg and slowly kneel down until your right knee touches the floor, lowering your hands to the floor at the same time to ease you into the posture. Balancing, clasp your hands in the same way as you did for the Eagle posture on the preceding page. Hold. Rise up and now go down on the opposite knee.

In a more advanced version of the pose, the hand gesture is taken first, and, with one foot raised, you slowly kneel down onto the opposite knee.

The name of the posture comes from the resemblance between the folded shape of the foot and a horse's head.

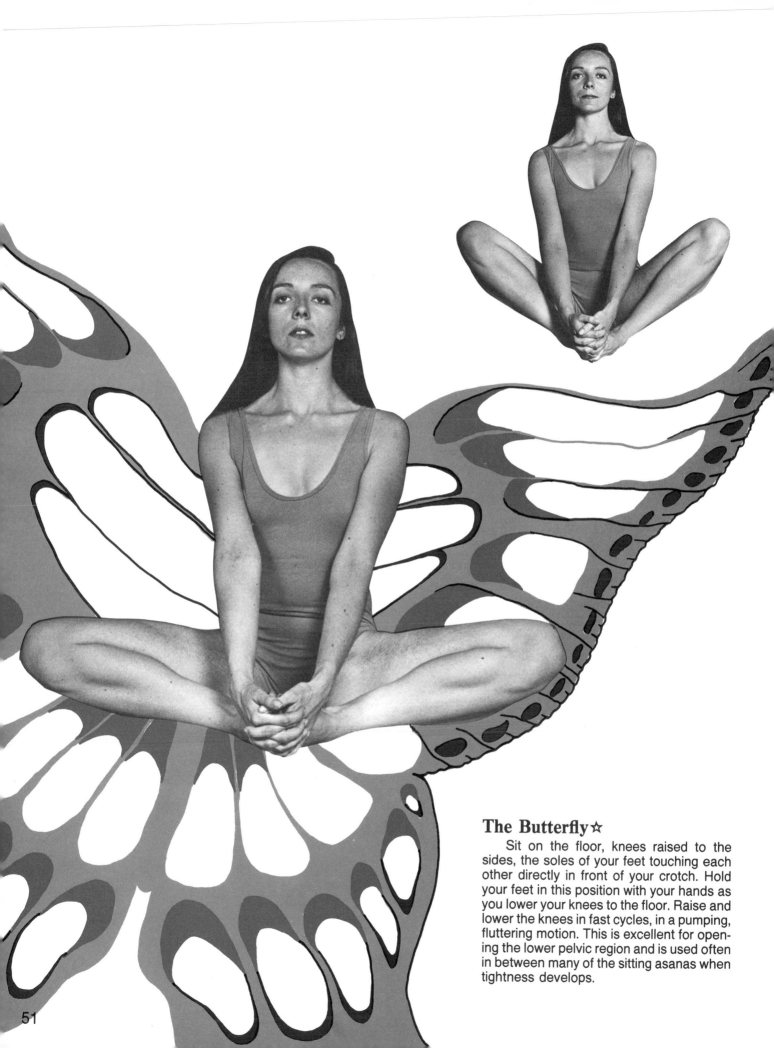

The Butterfly ☆

Sit on the floor, knees raised to the sides, the soles of your feet touching each other directly in front of your crotch. Hold your feet in this position with your hands as you lower your knees to the floor. Raise and lower the knees in fast cycles, in a pumping, fluttering motion. This is excellent for opening the lower pelvic region and is used often in between many of the sitting asanas when tightness develops.

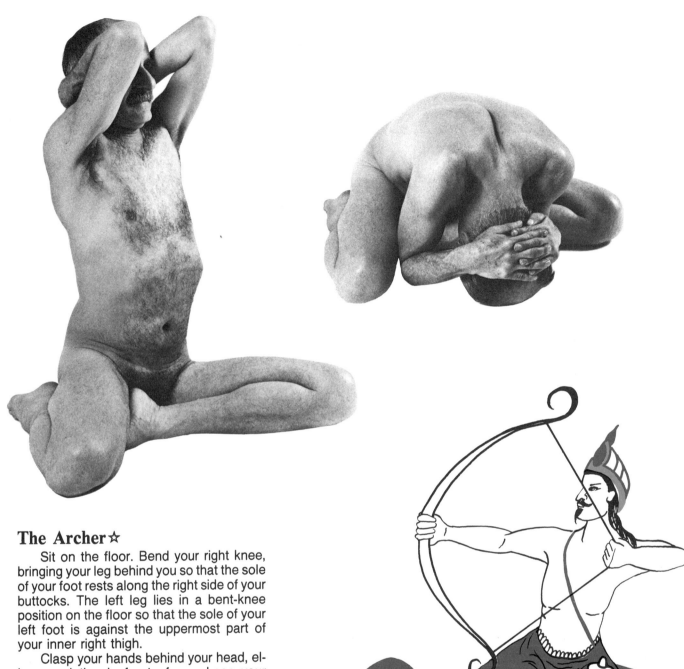

The Archer ☆

Sit on the floor. Bend your right knee, bringing your leg behind you so that the sole of your foot rests along the right side of your buttocks. The left leg lies in a bent-knee position on the floor so that the sole of your left foot is against the uppermost part of your inner right thigh.

Clasp your hands behind your head, elbows pointing in front of you. Lean your body forward toward the floor, head down, until your elbows touch the ground. Then slowly walk your elbows in toward your body, until your head rests on the floor. Hold and then slowly rise up.

Do the posture 2 more times; reverse your leg position and do the asana 3 more times. This is excellent for toning back and neck muscles.

The posture derives its name from the special manner in which archer–warriors sat on the floors of large wooden combat carts. Pulled by horses, the carts rumbled roughly across the landscape, doing battle. To steady himself while shooting, the crouching bowman wrapped his bent leg around a carved wooden post which protruded from the floor.

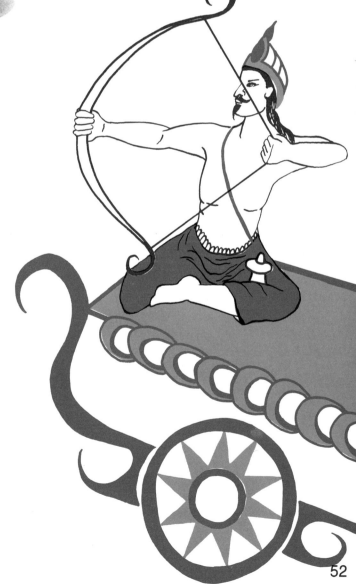

52

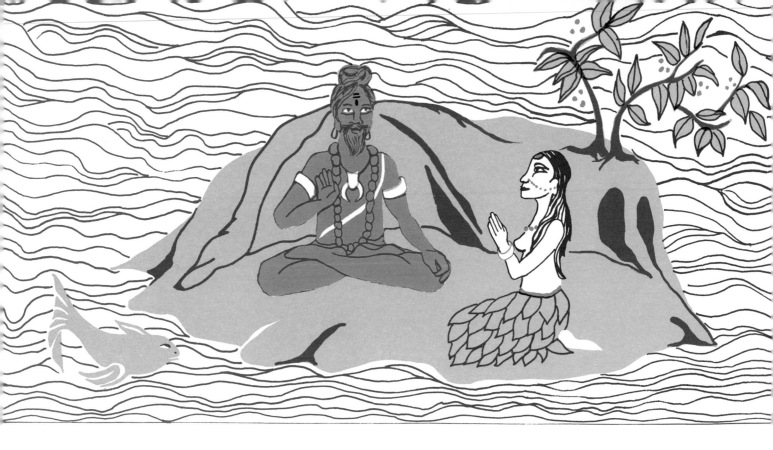

Sitting on an island in the upper Ganges, the god Shiva tells his consort, Parvati, the complete knowledges of yoga, the secrets and disciplines, the thousands of practices which will lead to liberation.

Parvati listens attentively, absorbing all the wonderful knowledges. A fish, in the water at the shore's edge, listens too, equally attentive.

Shiva notices the fish, his particular quality of intense attention, his discipline and stillness as he listens. Impressed by his nature, he honors him by making him a man and then gives him the task of being the Father of Yoga and spreading the knowledges he has been privileged to hear. Matsya means fish in Sanscrit, Matsyendra is the name of the Father of Yoga.

☆ The Simple Spinal Twist *Matsyendrasana*

Raise your left leg bending it at the knee, cross over the right leg and place your foot on the floor next to the right knee. Place your right arm around the outside of your raised knee, grasping the inside of your ankle with your hand. Keep your right leg firmly on the floor.

Twist the body backward looking over your left shoulder. Place your left arm behind your back, bent at the elbow. Your left hand, palm facing outward, rests on your right hip. Repeat the asana, reversing the position.

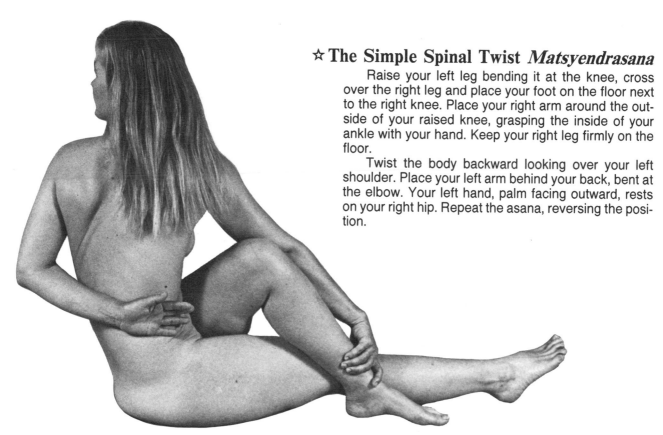

53

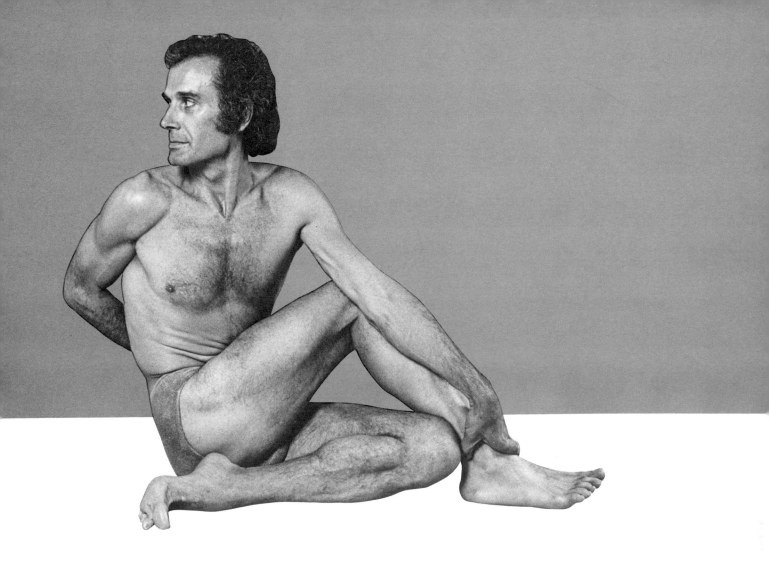

The Classic Spinal Twist

Sit on the floor, feet straight in front of you. Raise your right leg at the knee, cross the right foot over your extended leg and place it on the floor next to the left knee. Curve your left leg around your body so that the foot rests against the right side of your buttocks. The left arm comes around the outside of the right knee and the hand grabs onto the ankle.

Twist the body backwards looking over your right shoulder. Place the right arm behind your back, bent at the elbow; the right hand, palm facing outward rests on the left hip.

Hold the position while doing light breathing. Relax. Repeat the posture reversing the position of the arms and legs to twist the spine to the opposite side.

This asana is a wonderful exercise for the spine and all the ligaments, nerves and blood vessels moving to and from it.

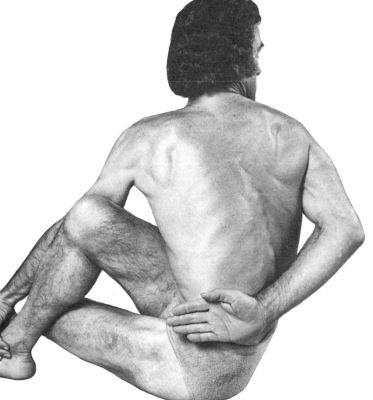

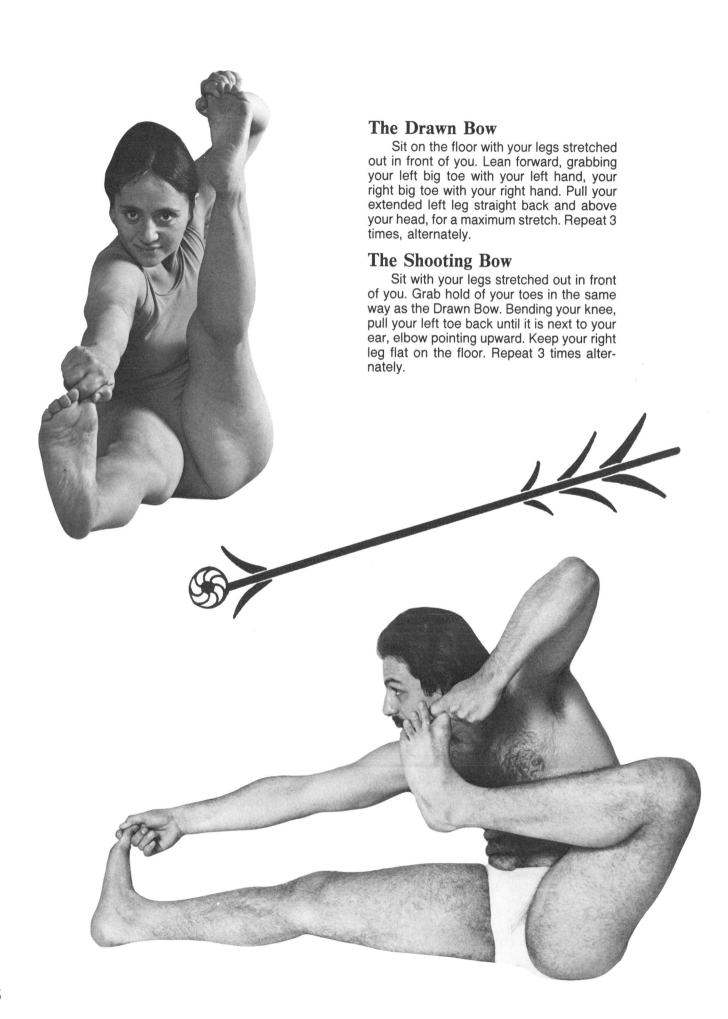

The Drawn Bow

Sit on the floor with your legs stretched out in front of you. Lean forward, grabbing your left big toe with your left hand, your right big toe with your right hand. Pull your extended left leg straight back and above your head, for a maximum stretch. Repeat 3 times, alternately.

The Shooting Bow

Sit with your legs stretched out in front of you. Grab hold of your toes in the same way as the Drawn Bow. Bending your knee, pull your left toe back until it is next to your ear, elbow pointing upward. Keep your right leg flat on the floor. Repeat 3 times alternately.

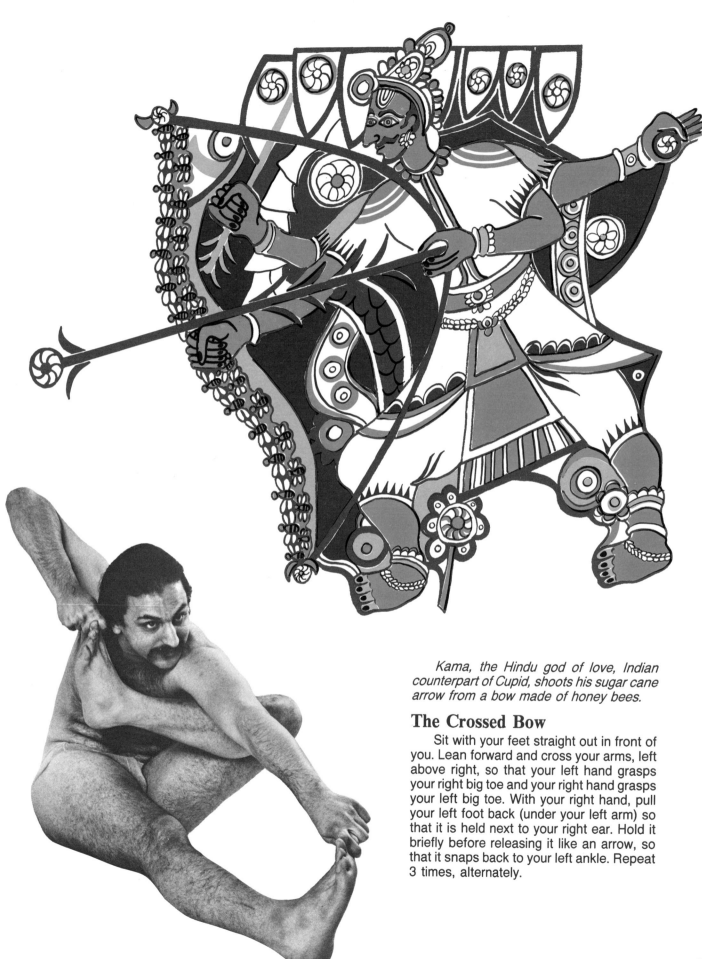

Kama, the Hindu god of love, Indian counterpart of Cupid, shoots his sugar cane arrow from a bow made of honey bees.

The Crossed Bow

Sit with your feet straight out in front of you. Lean forward and cross your arms, left above right, so that your left hand grasps your right big toe and your right hand grasps your left big toe. With your right hand, pull your left foot back (under your left arm) so that it is held next to your right ear. Hold it briefly before releasing it like an arrow, so that it snaps back to your left ankle. Repeat 3 times, alternately.

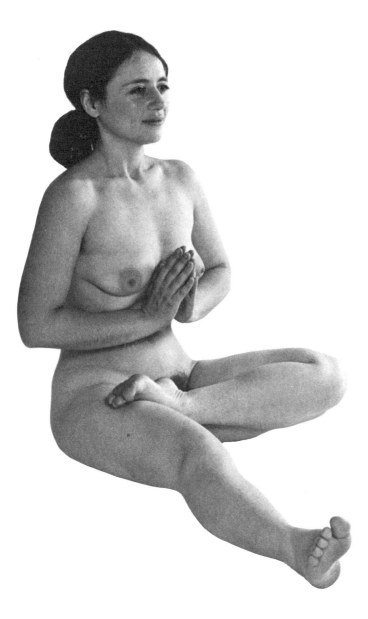

The Head-to-Knee Bend *Shirsa Janu*

Sit on the floor, both legs extended in front of you, your back straight. Fold your left leg over your right, resting your foot on your upper right thigh. Put your hands to your chest, palms together.

Raise your hands above your head, bring them down to your chest again and slowly bend forward, placing your clasped hands on your right knee, head resting on top of your hands. Hold, then lift your torso. Raise your hands up over your head and repeat the cycle once more.

When you lower the body for the third time, bend forward and place both hands around your extended right foot. Bring your elbows to the ground, your head touching your right knee. Rise up and do this series on the other side, changing leg positions.

This is an especially good stretch for the upper and lower back.

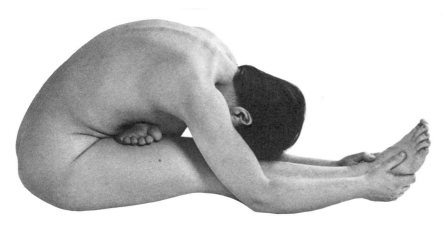

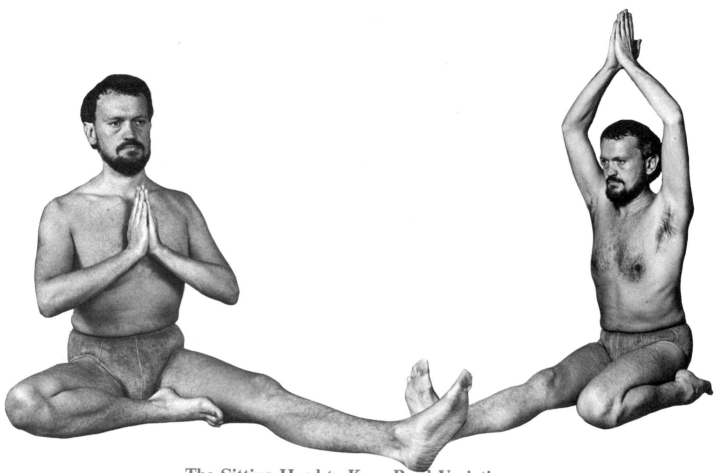

The Sitting Head-to-Knee Bend Variations

Sit on the floor, both legs extended in front of you. Take the sole of your right foot and place it on the inside of your left thigh at the crotch. Put your hands on your chest, palms together, raise the hands above your head and then bring them back to the chest. Lean forward touching your hands to your knee, head resting on top of your hands. Do this twice and then lean all the way forward grasping your feet, head to the knee.

Slowly rise up and repeat on the other side, changing your foot position.

Do the same routine as the previous posture, only this time fold one leg at the knee, wrapping it around the outside of the thigh, heel to the buttocks. After 3 rounds, reverse the foot position and do the asana again.

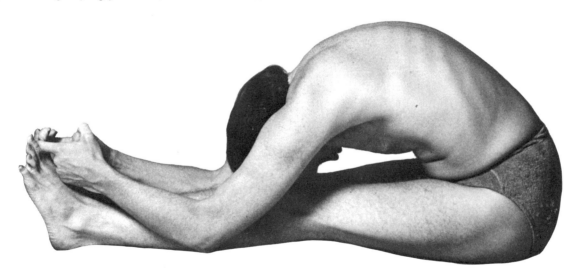

The Full Head-to-Knee Bend *Paschimothan*

Extend your feet straight out in front of you. Exhaling, slowly lean forward and catch hold of your big toes; the elbows touch the floor, your head is buried between your legs. Hold out the breath. Inhaling, slowly rise up. Now hold in the breath, then relax.

One of the important classic asanas. Besides strengthening the muscles in the calf and behind the knee, it stimulates the entire abdominal area—such organs as the kidney, liver and pancreas.

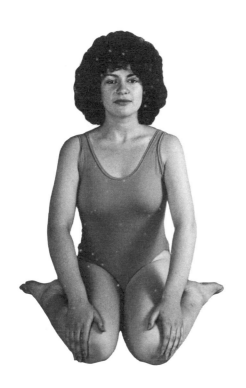

The Hero

Sit in the Thunderbolt posture. Rise up on your knees and spread your legs so that when you sit down again you will be sitting between your feet.

From this position slowly lean backward, balancing on your elbows until your head touches the floor. Lift your hands to your chest, palms touching. Your head is arched back, holding the weight of the body; the back is in a high curve. Beginners should do this posture slowly. It puts a lot of stress on the pelvis, back and legs, but when mastered, it exercises these parts thoroughly.

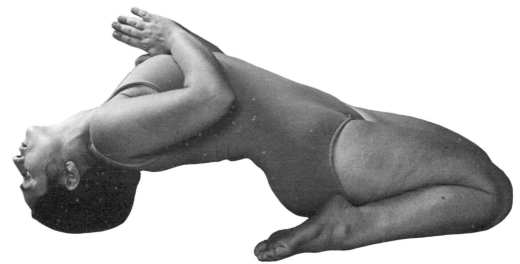

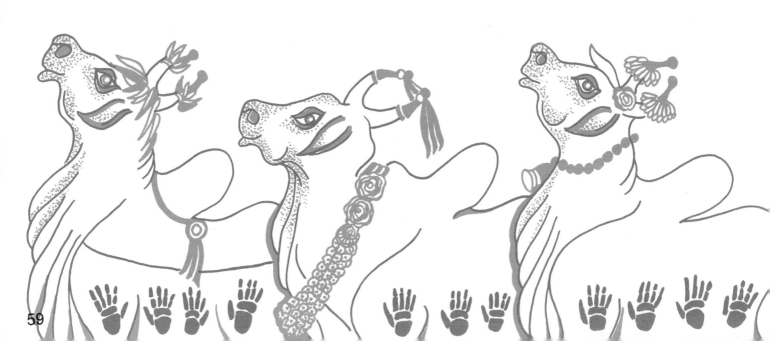

The Cow *Gomhukasana*

Sit in the Thunderbolt posture. Rise up and spread your legs so that you now sit down between them. Raise your right hand up and over your shoulder onto your back, palm facing inward. Bring your left hand down and behind the back, palm facing outward, and then move it up to lock fingers with the right hand.

Slowly bend forward and touch your head to your left knee. Swing the head to the right knee and then rise up again, fingers clasped, elbow in the air. Do this 2 more times. Now reverse the hand position and do 3 more rounds.

This asana stretches the shoulder joints and rib cage and exercises the knee and ankle joints. Develop the sitting part of this asana slowly, since it may take a while to spread your ankles and sit between your feet.

The Indian cow, a special breed with a large hump at the top of his back, we call a Brahman (the highest of cows). Never slaughtered, he has a distinct place in the psyche of Indian society. He is connected with Shiva, being his vehicle and sometimes his embodiment. All Shiva temples have a sculpture outside of the venerated cow pointing toward the entrance. Some of these can be quite elaborate and beautiful like this carved stone statue in Mysore, which is almost sixty feet high.

On different festival days real cows are painted and festooned.

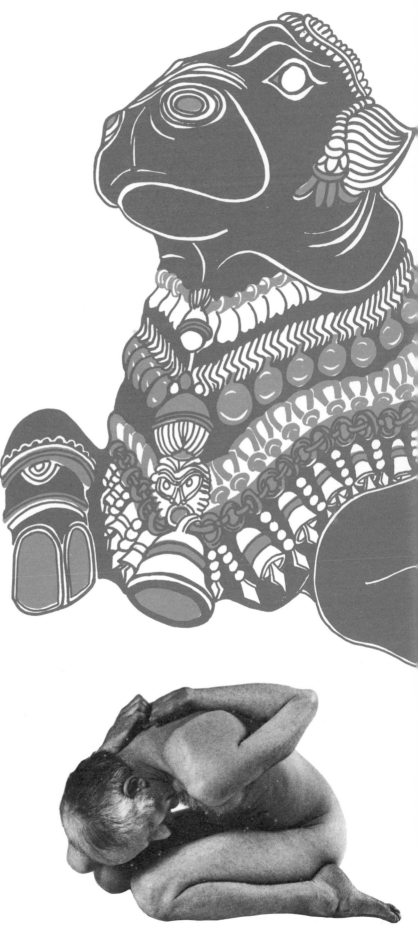

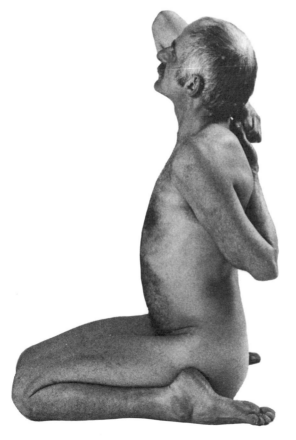

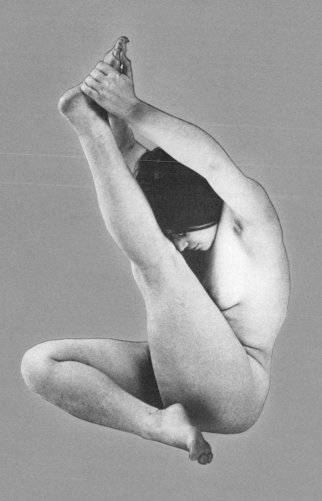

The Side Leg Swing

Sit on the floor. Curve your right leg along the floor in front of you so that the heel of your right foot is next to your upper left thigh. By bending your knee, bring your left thigh close to your chest; the sole of your foot is flat on the floor. Slip your fingers under your arch and slowly lift your left leg straight up toward your head. Tucking your chin under, bring your forehead forward to meet your raised knee. Hold the position.

Now slowly swing your right arm to your right side as you lift your head and bring the held left leg to the opposite side. Both arms should be completely extended at shoulder level and parallel to the floor. Hold for several seconds before returning to the forehead-to-knee position and then back to the floor.

Reverse the position and now swing your right leg to the side. This posture releases any tension in the lower back and pelvic area while toning the thighs.

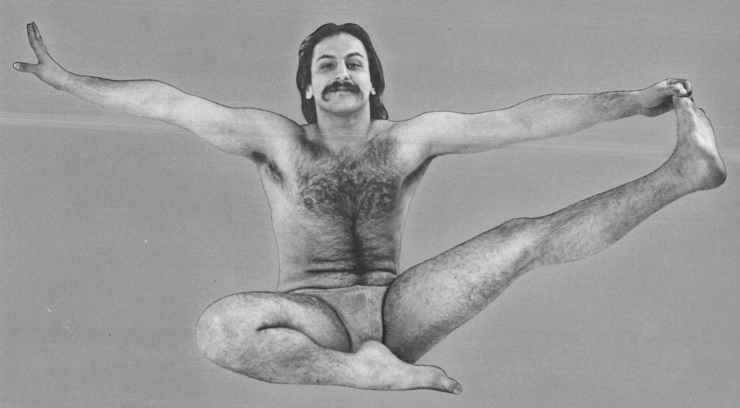

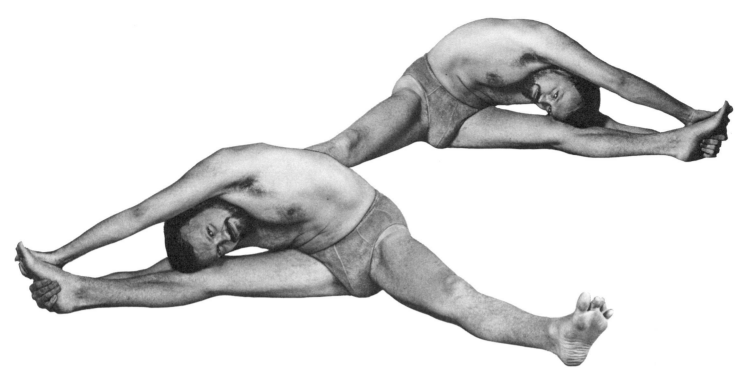

Sitting Side Bends

Sit on the floor with your legs spread apart as wide as possible. Keep your knees straight and legs flat against the floor. Bring your right hand around the outside of your right leg to grab onto the sole of your foot. Lift your left hand over your head as you exhale and bend the right side of your body down to lie on top of your leg. Grab hold of your toes with your left hand.

The side of your head should rest on top of your knee as you hold the posture. Inhaling, lift your arm and then your body back to the sitting position. Bend 2 more times to your right side before repeating the bend to the opposite side for 3 more rounds.

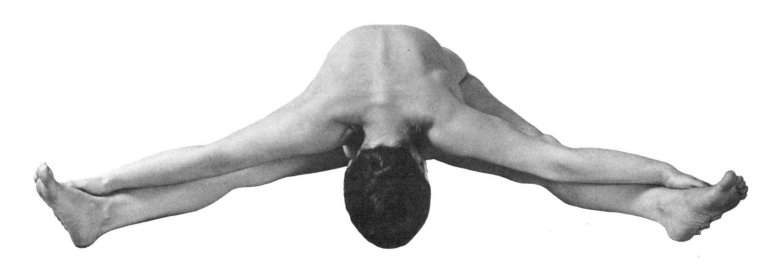

Sitting Front Bend

With your legs spread wide apart, bring your hands around the outside of your legs so that you can grab hold of the soles of your feet. Slowly bend forward until your forehead touches the ground. Hold for a few seconds before lifting back into the sitting position. Do this frontal bend twice more.

You can feel the work this posture is doing for your thighs the very first time you try it.

The Turtle *Kurmasana*

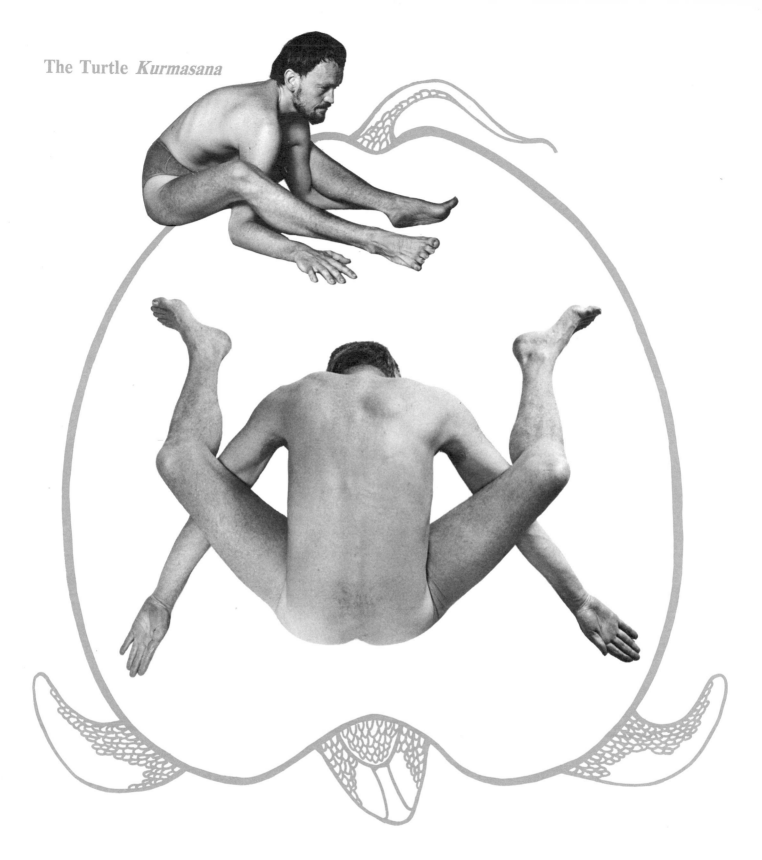

Sit on the floor. Your legs extend in front of you, feet spread about two feet apart. Lift your knees upward toward your chest so that the soles of your feet are flat on the floor. Now put your hands between your bent legs, through the space created by your raised knees.

Lower your torso forward as you stretch your arms out to the side in a horizontal line on the floor. Touch your chin or forehead to the floor in front of you.

Twist your hands so that your palms are facing upward and slide your outstretched arms along the floor to point behind you. Now lower your knees so that your body, arms and legs are as flat to the floor as possible. You can hold this position for up to a minute.

This posture is held in high esteem by yogis who find its effects bring stillness and equanimity to the mind and body. Physically it activates the organs of the abdomen and strengthens the spine.

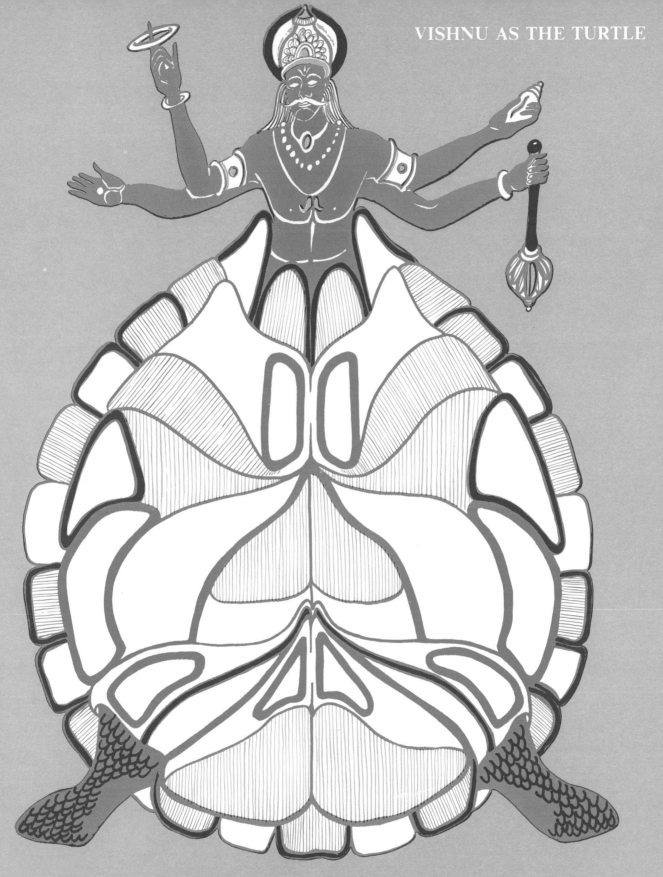

This asana is named after Vishnu as the turtle, another one of the evolutionary developments of man mirrored in the different forms of the god Vishnu.

During the time of the flooding of the universe, many divine treasures were lost and Vishnu turned himself into a tortoise so he could dive to the bottom of the all-encompassing ocean to recover them. A simple churn was also invented, using a holy mountain on his back as a churning stick and a divine snake for the twirling rope. The oceans were churned and churned and the lost treasures, including Vishnu's consort, Lakshmi, were spun into existence again.

The tortoise in his shell is a symbol for the yogi, whose senses are withdrawn from the outer world into inner contemplation.

The Bow *Danurasana*

Lie on your stomach resting your chin or forehead on the floor. By bending your knees up and stretching your hands behind you, grab hold of your ankles with your hands. Exhale all of the breath from your lungs by forcefully spitting it out of your mouth in a single gust.

Now lift your head back, chest high off the floor. At the same time raise your knees and pelvis high into the air. Your arms act like a tightening string to make your body taut as a bent bow.

All of the weight of your body should be resting only on your abdomen. With no air in the lungs, gently rock back and forth on the floor several times, from the point of your lower rib cage to the pelvic bones. Release your legs and relax back to the floor.

The internal viscera of the abdominal area are gently massaged, increasing your digestive powers.

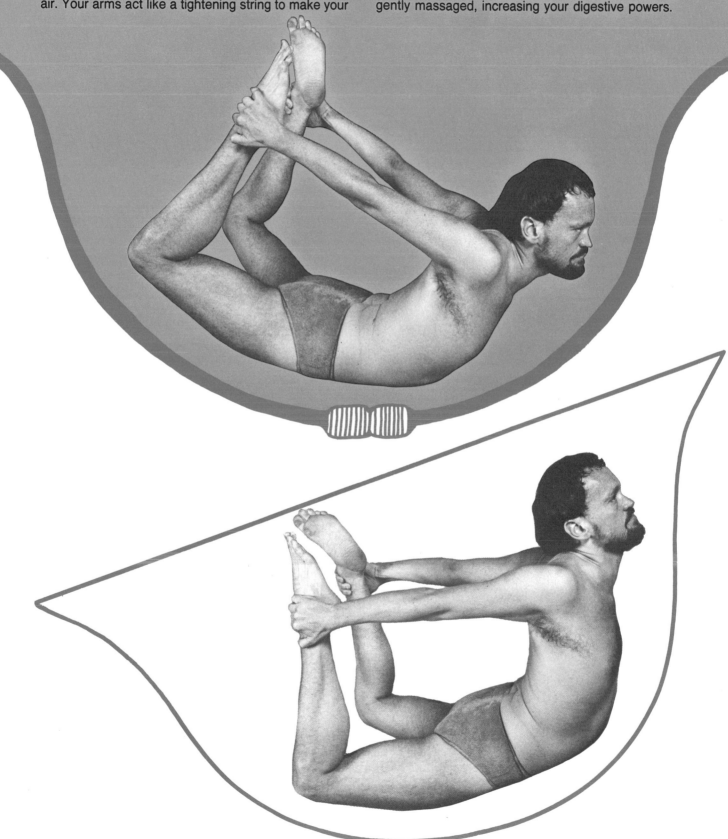

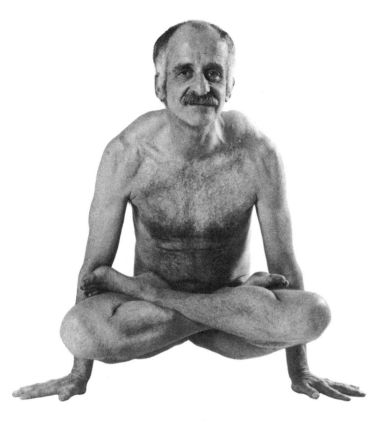

The Floating Lotus

Sit in the Full Lotus posture. Put the flat of your hands on the floor, just outside of your upper thighs. Push down on your hands as you lift your locked feet off the floor. Hold the posture for as long as is comfortable and then let yourself down. On the next lift try to raise up higher and sustain the pose longer.

In another variation, to further strengthen the arms, swing yourself back and forth while suspended above your hands.

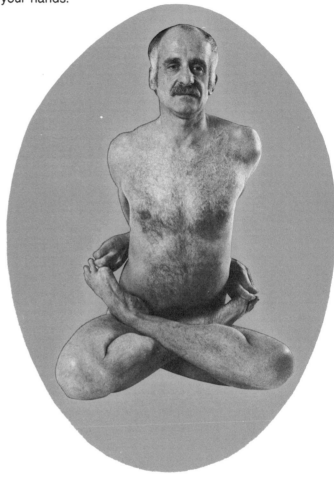

The Bound Lotus

Sit in the Lotus posture, with your feet as far back on your thighs as possible, toes pointing backward. Cross your arms behind your back, lean forward slightly for flexibility and grab your right toe with your right hand and your left toe with your left hand. Sit up as straight as you can. Hold.

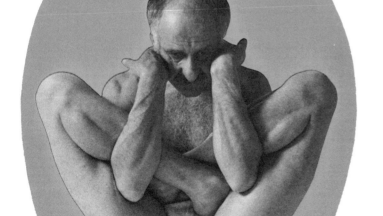

The Fetus

Sit in the Lotus posture. Raise your knees, balancing on your tailbone as you place your hands through the folds under your knees until the arms have gone through the space, up to the elbow. Now fold the arm at the elbow, bringing the hands back towards the head. Incline the head slightly forward to permit the hands to hold the head at the temples. Hold the pose, balanced on your tailbone.

In this pose, circulation of blood in the abdominal region is stimulated, since the area is fully contracted.

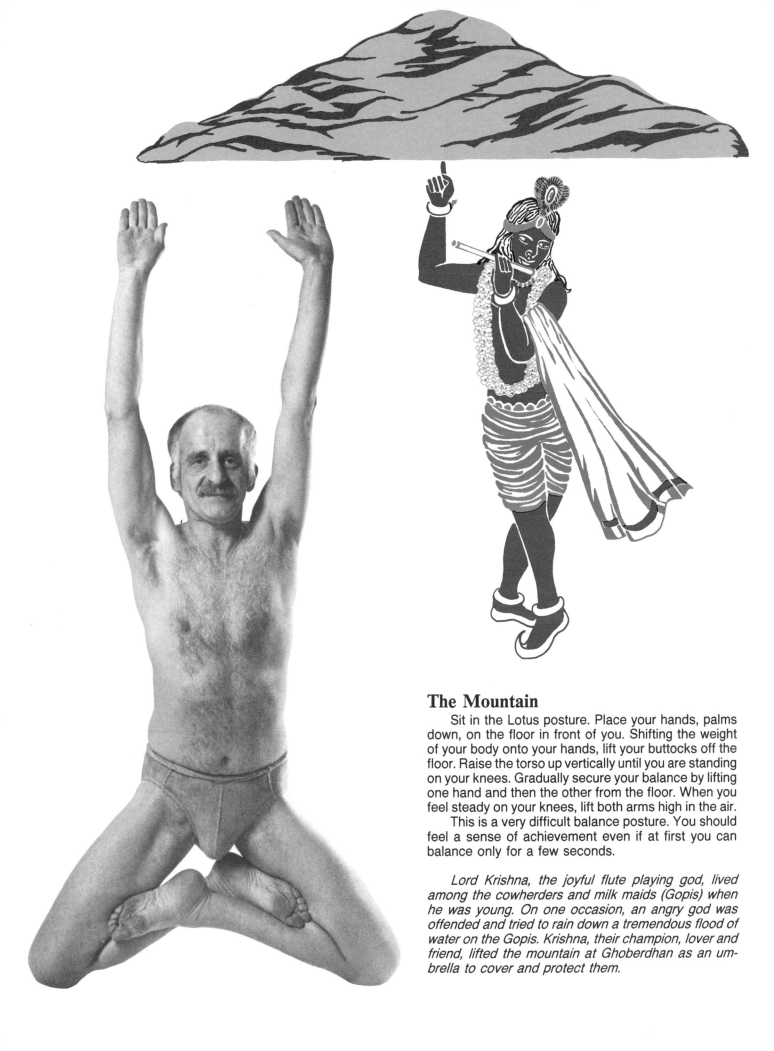

The Mountain

Sit in the Lotus posture. Place your hands, palms down, on the floor in front of you. Shifting the weight of your body onto your hands, lift your buttocks off the floor. Raise the torso up vertically until you are standing on your knees. Gradually secure your balance by lifting one hand and then the other from the floor. When you feel steady on your knees, lift both arms high in the air.

This is a very difficult balance posture. You should feel a sense of achievement even if at first you can balance only for a few seconds.

Lord Krishna, the joyful flute playing god, lived among the cowherders and milk maids (Gopis) when he was young. On one occasion, an angry god was offended and tried to rain down a tremendous flood of water on the Gopis. Krishna, their champion, lover and friend, lifted the mountain at Ghoberdhan as an umbrella to cover and protect them.

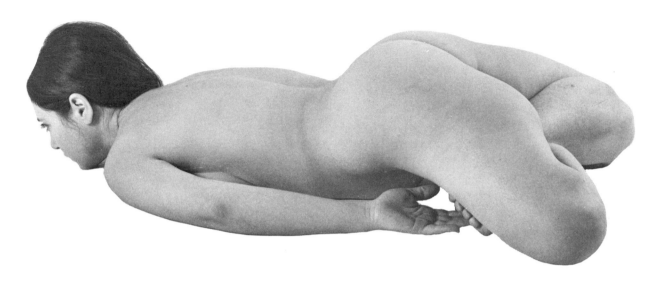

Over-the-Lotus Bend

Sit in the Lotus posture. Place your hands on the floor in front of you. Rest the weight of your body on your hands as you lift the buttocks and lean your body forward. Walk your hands forward so that you are balanced in an all-fours position on top of your knees and hands.

Bend your elbows and lower your body to the floor so that you are lying on your stomach and over your folded legs. Rest your head on your chin. Your arms should lie next to your sides. Hold this position for a minute before lifting the body back into the sitting position.

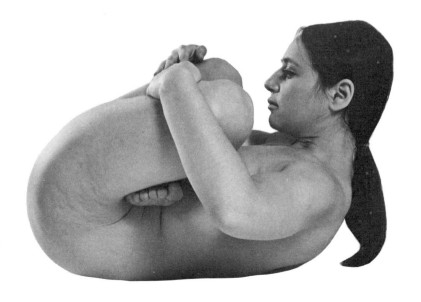

Head-to-Lotus Bend

Lie with your back flat on the floor. Fold your legs into the Lotus posture. Bend the Lotus toward your body. Placing your hands around the outside of your thighs, pull your chest and head forward as close to your legs as possible. Hold for several seconds before relaxing back to the floor.

Do this posture 2 more times.

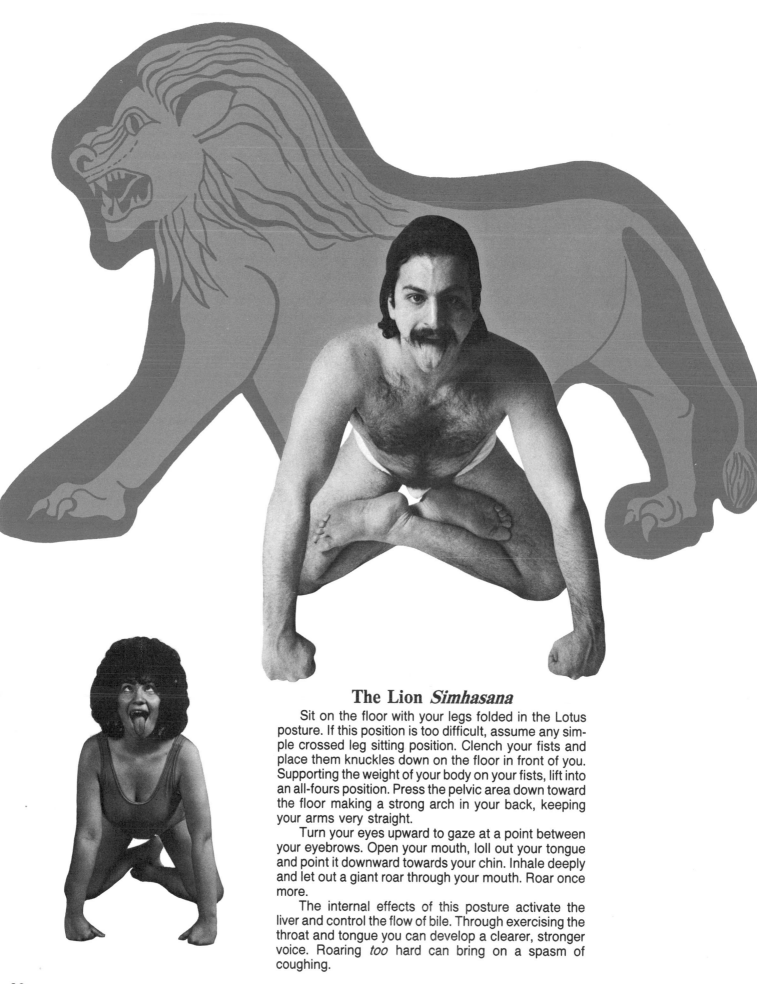

The Lion *Simhasana*

Sit on the floor with your legs folded in the Lotus posture. If this position is too difficult, assume any simple crossed leg sitting position. Clench your fists and place them knuckles down on the floor in front of you. Supporting the weight of your body on your fists, lift into an all-fours position. Press the pelvic area down toward the floor making a strong arch in your back, keeping your arms very straight.

Turn your eyes upward to gaze at a point between your eyebrows. Open your mouth, loll out your tongue and point it downward towards your chin. Inhale deeply and let out a giant roar through your mouth. Roar once more.

The internal effects of this posture activate the liver and control the flow of bile. Through exercising the throat and tongue you can develop a clearer, stronger voice. Roaring *too* hard can bring on a spasm of coughing.

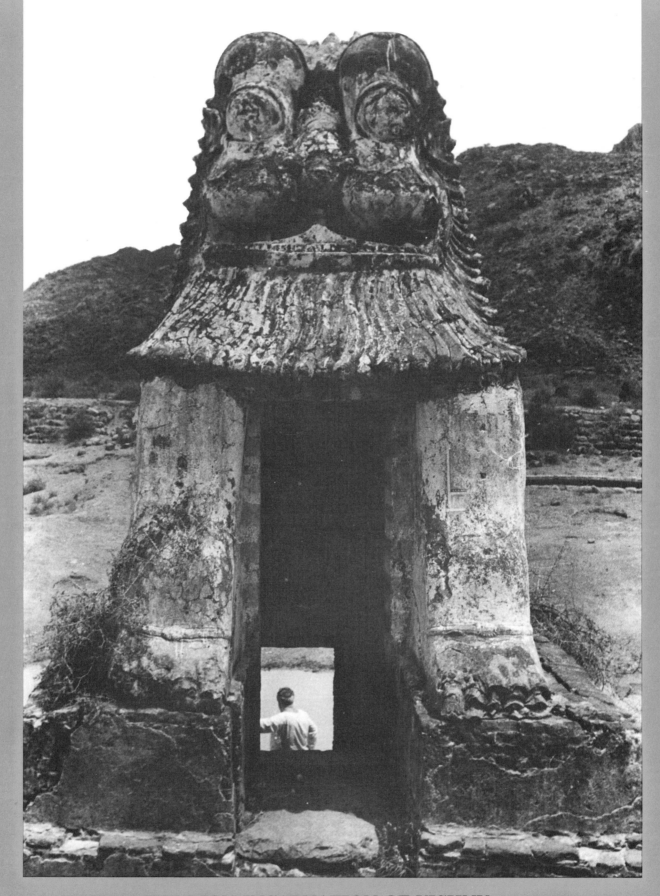

THE LION INCARNATION OF VISHNU

The lion, incarnation of Lord Vishnu, is often depicted in Indian sculpture. This stone lion stands on the side of the road to Tanjor in southern India. A stairway descends inside of him leading to a small lake below. He has been standing in Simhasana for over five hundred years.

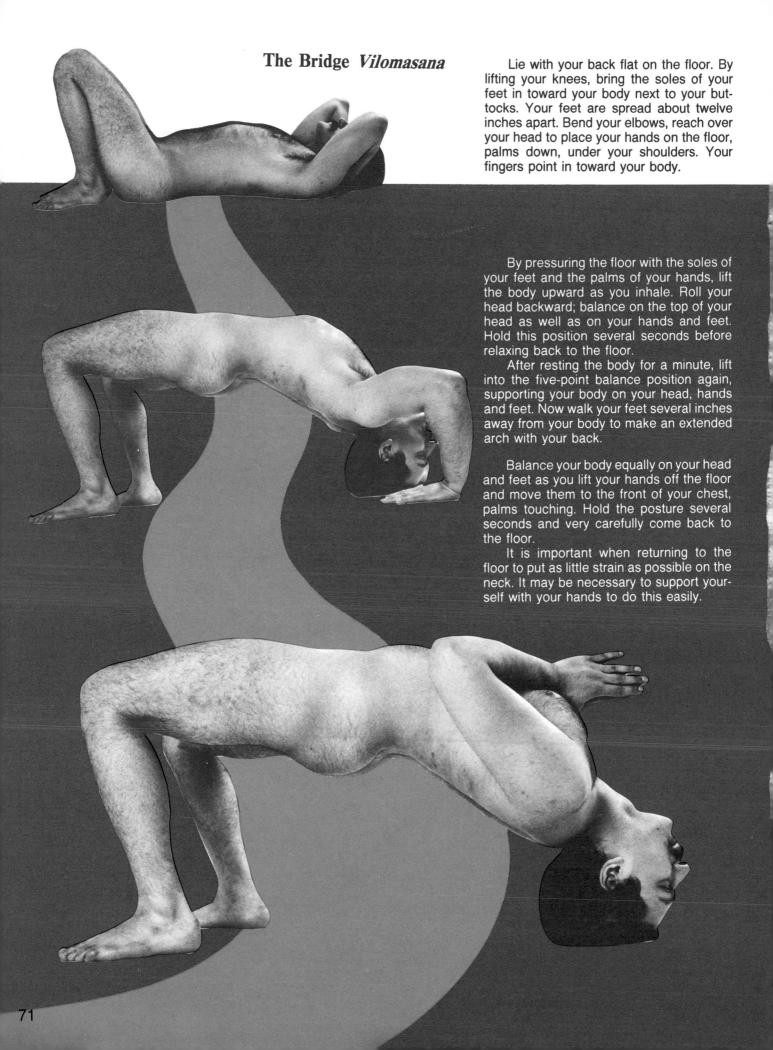

The Bridge *Vilomasana*

Lie with your back flat on the floor. By lifting your knees, bring the soles of your feet in toward your body next to your buttocks. Your feet are spread about twelve inches apart. Bend your elbows, reach over your head to place your hands on the floor, palms down, under your shoulders. Your fingers point in toward your body.

By pressuring the floor with the soles of your feet and the palms of your hands, lift the body upward as you inhale. Roll your head backward; balance on the top of your head as well as on your hands and feet. Hold this position several seconds before relaxing back to the floor.

After resting the body for a minute, lift into the five-point balance position again, supporting your body on your head, hands and feet. Now walk your feet several inches away from your body to make an extended arch with your back.

Balance your body equally on your head and feet as you lift your hands off the floor and move them to the front of your chest, palms touching. Hold the posture several seconds and very carefully come back to the floor.

It is important when returning to the floor to put as little strain as possible on the neck. It may be necessary to support yourself with your hands to do this easily.

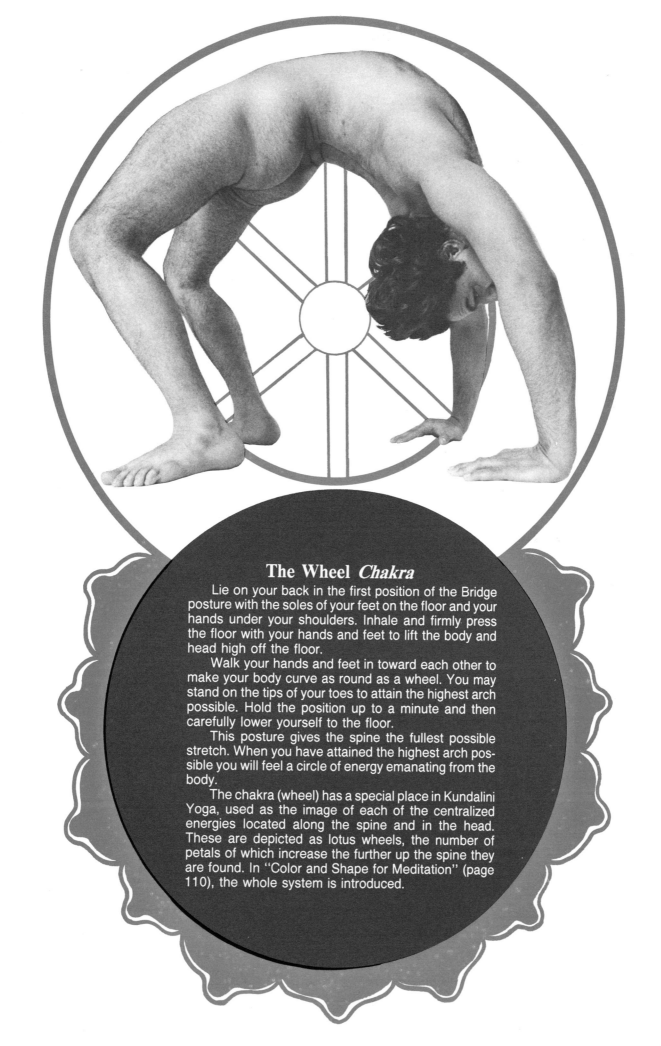

The Wheel *Chakra*

Lie on your back in the first position of the Bridge posture with the soles of your feet on the floor and your hands under your shoulders. Inhale and firmly press the floor with your hands and feet to lift the body and head high off the floor.

Walk your hands and feet in toward each other to make your body curve as round as a wheel. You may stand on the tips of your toes to attain the highest arch possible. Hold the position up to a minute and then carefully lower yourself to the floor.

This posture gives the spine the fullest possible stretch. When you have attained the highest arch possible you will feel a circle of energy emanating from the body.

The chakra (wheel) has a special place in Kundalini Yoga, used as the image of each of the centralized energies located along the spine and in the head. These are depicted as lotus wheels, the number of petals of which increase the further up the spine they are found. In "Color and Shape for Meditation" (page 110), the whole system is introduced.

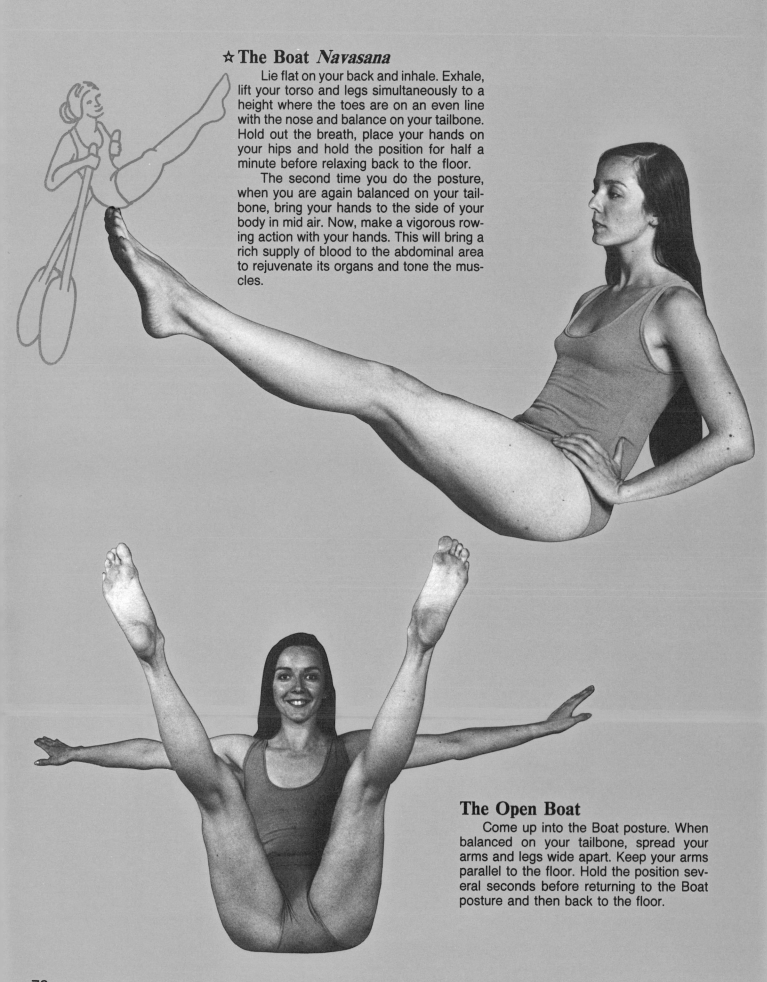

☆ The Boat *Navasana*

Lie flat on your back and inhale. Exhale, lift your torso and legs simultaneously to a height where the toes are on an even line with the nose and balance on your tailbone. Hold out the breath, place your hands on your hips and hold the position for half a minute before relaxing back to the floor.

The second time you do the posture, when you are again balanced on your tailbone, bring your hands to the side of your body in mid air. Now, make a vigorous rowing action with your hands. This will bring a rich supply of blood to the abdominal area to rejuvenate its organs and tone the muscles.

The Open Boat

Come up into the Boat posture. When balanced on your tailbone, spread your arms and legs wide apart. Keep your arms parallel to the floor. Hold the position several seconds before returning to the Boat posture and then back to the floor.

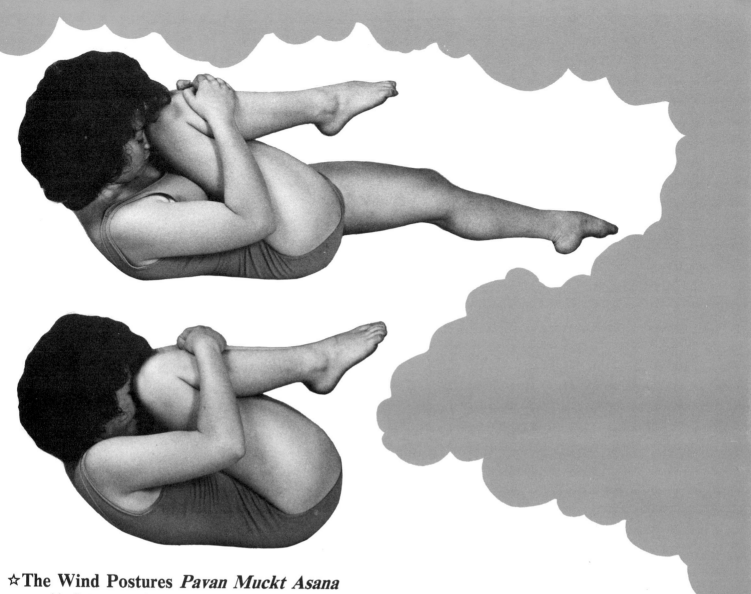

☆ The Wind Postures *Pavan Muckt Asana*

Lie flat on your back, hands at your sides. Inhale as you bend your right knee, bringing the upper thigh to lie on top of your chest. Wrap your hands around your raised leg and lift your forehead to touch the knee. Exhale forcefully, spitting the air out of your mouth as you quickly spring your leg back to the floor. Repeat the exercise, raising and then releasing the left leg.

Now, raise both knees to your chest. Wrap your hands around your raised legs, lift your forehead to touch your knees and then spring both legs back to the floor using the same breathing pattern as before.

This posture helps to relieve any gas in the stomach and is also used to tone the abdominal area.

☆ The Slab

This posture can be used to balance the effects of any forward bending position.

Sit on the floor, legs extended in front of you. Place your hands a few inches behind you along the outside of your buttocks. Your fingers point in the opposite direction to the body. By pressing the palms of your hands against the floor, lift your body into the air to make a diagonal line from head to toe. The soles of your feet should be flat on the floor, the toes pointing straight ahead. Hold and relax back to the floor.

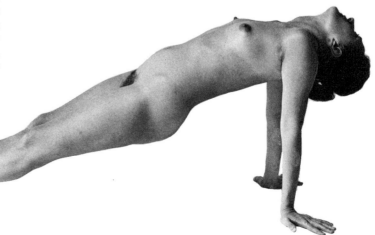

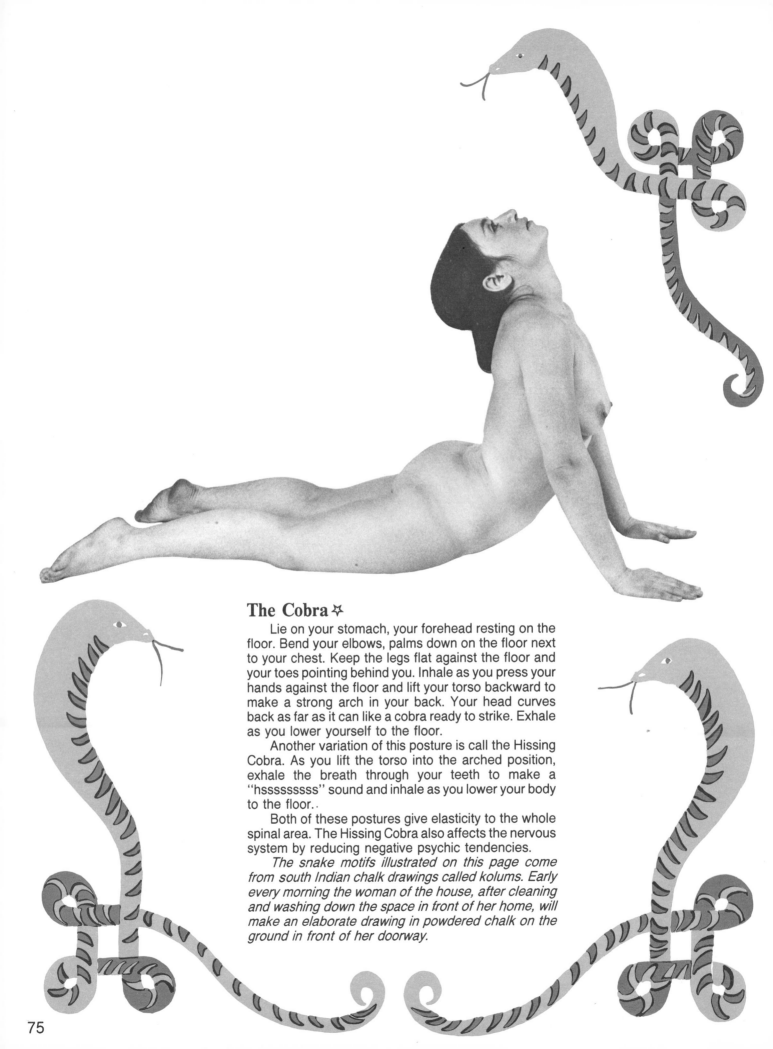

The Cobra ✧

Lie on your stomach, your forehead resting on the floor. Bend your elbows, palms down on the floor next to your chest. Keep the legs flat against the floor and your toes pointing behind you. Inhale as you press your hands against the floor and lift your torso backward to make a strong arch in your back. Your head curves back as far as it can like a cobra ready to strike. Exhale as you lower yourself to the floor.

Another variation of this posture is call the Hissing Cobra. As you lift the torso into the arched position, exhale the breath through your teeth to make a "hsssssssss" sound and inhale as you lower your body to the floor.

Both of these postures give elasticity to the whole spinal area. The Hissing Cobra also affects the nervous system by reducing negative psychic tendencies.

The snake motifs illustrated on this page come from south Indian chalk drawings called kolums. Early every morning the woman of the house, after cleaning and washing down the space in front of her home, will make an elaborate drawing in powdered chalk on the ground in front of her doorway.

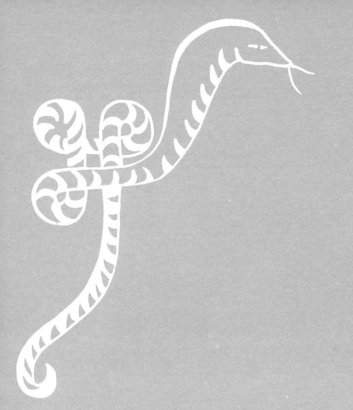

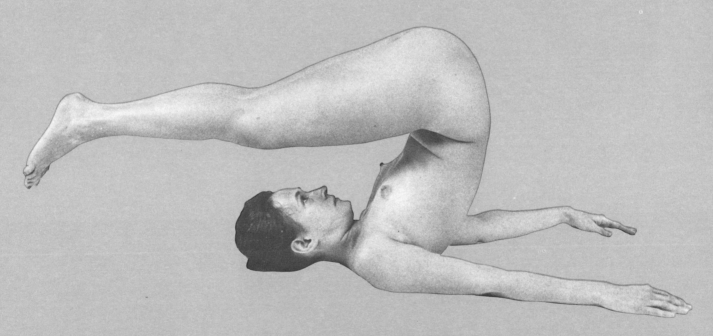

The Parallel-Floor Posture

Lie on your back, hands at your sides, palms on the floor. On the in-breath, slowly raise both legs straight up in the air. Exhale as you press down on your hands and raise your buttocks off the floor. Slowly bring your feet over your head so the legs are parallel to the floor. Hold. Inhale as you bring your feet straight up into the air again, exhale as you carefully lower your buttocks and feet.

When descending from various postures onto your back, always move very slowly, feeling each vertebra move back into place. The spine is our most flexible bone structure, but it can easily be twisted or pulled.

To become more conscious of the spine and its parts, do this special exercise.

Stand erect, hands in front of you. Breathe slowly, in and out. Lean your head forward slightly, feeling the first vertebra in the top of your back tilt.

Breathe in and out concentrating the flow of breath on that area. Lean your head forward a little more, now bending the second vertebra. Breathe in and out of that area.

Continue to bend forward very, very slowly, with a breath for each vertebra, letting your arms drop forward. When you have released the whole neck and back, start slowly rising up again in the same manner. There are 33 vertebra in the spine.

Single and Double Knee-Bend

Lift into the Shoulder Stand. Bring your right knee down to touch your forehead by sliding the sole of your foot along your left leg. Hold for up to a minute before bending the left knee to the forehead in the same way. After bringing each knee to the forehead separately, bend both knees and slowly bring them down together to touch the forehead.

The right knee bend stimulates the liver; the left, the spleen. The double leg bend stimulates the pancreas.

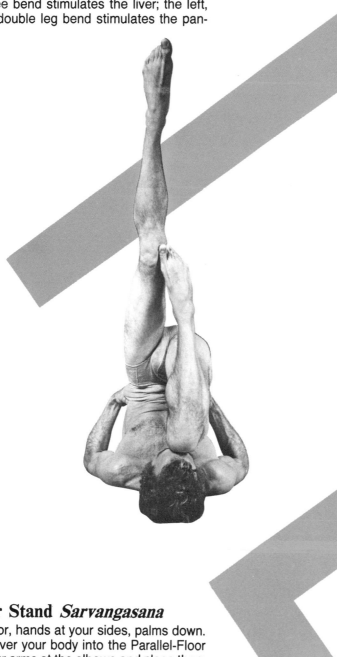

The Shoulder Stand *Sarvangasana*

Lie on the floor, hands at your sides, palms down. Raise your legs over your body into the Parallel-Floor posture. Bend your arms at the elbows and place them on the back against the lower rib cage to support yourself. Lift your legs straight up in the air and steady your torso with your hands. Your weight is held by your shoulders and arms. With the body in a vertical line to the floor, you are in the full Shoulder Stand.

Remain in this position from five to fifteen minutes according to your ability. Then release your hands and very slowly lower your back to the floor. Relax for several minutes after doing this pose.

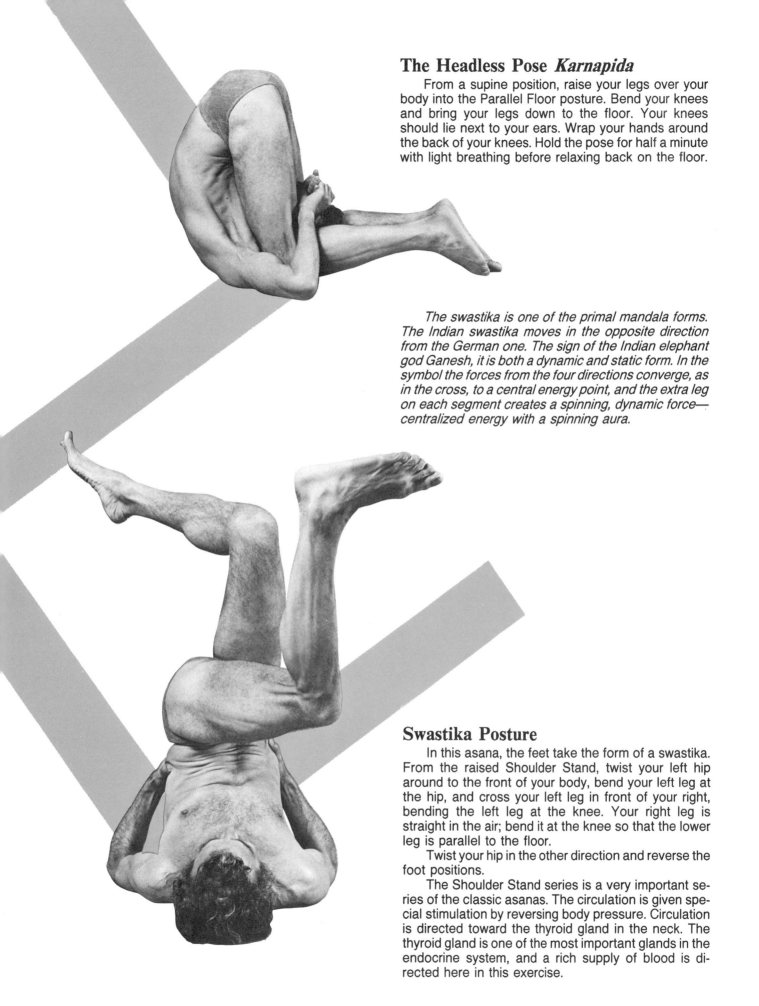

The Headless Pose *Karnapida*

From a supine position, raise your legs over your body into the Parallel Floor posture. Bend your knees and bring your legs down to the floor. Your knees should lie next to your ears. Wrap your hands around the back of your knees. Hold the pose for half a minute with light breathing before relaxing back on the floor.

The swastika is one of the primal mandala forms. The Indian swastika moves in the opposite direction from the German one. The sign of the Indian elephant god Ganesh, it is both a dynamic and static form. In the symbol the forces from the four directions converge, as in the cross, to a central energy point, and the extra leg on each segment creates a spinning, dynamic force— centralized energy with a spinning aura.

Swastika Posture

In this asana, the feet take the form of a swastika. From the raised Shoulder Stand, twist your left hip around to the front of your body, bend your left leg at the hip, and cross your left leg in front of your right, bending the left leg at the knee. Your right leg is straight in the air; bend it at the knee so that the lower leg is parallel to the floor.

Twist your hip in the other direction and reverse the foot positions.

The Shoulder Stand series is a very important series of the classic asanas. The circulation is given special stimulation by reversing body pressure. Circulation is directed toward the thyroid gland in the neck. The thyroid gland is one of the most important glands in the endocrine system, and a rich supply of blood is directed here in this exercise.

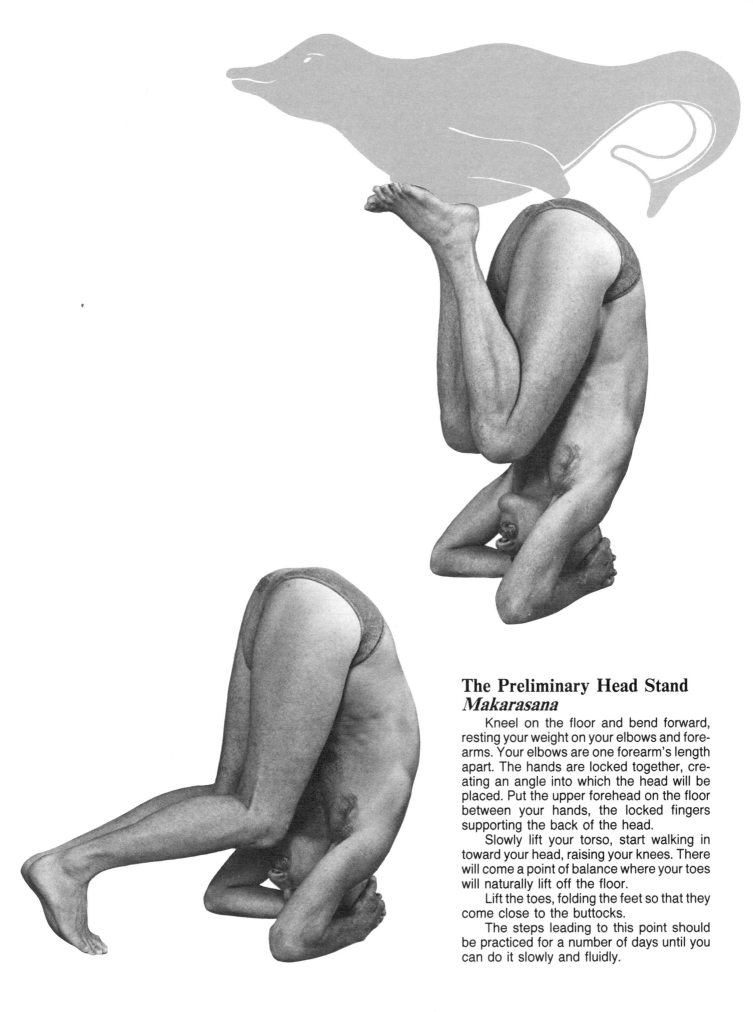

The Preliminary Head Stand
Makarasana

Kneel on the floor and bend forward, resting your weight on your elbows and forearms. Your elbows are one forearm's length apart. The hands are locked together, creating an angle into which the head will be placed. Put the upper forehead on the floor between your hands, the locked fingers supporting the back of the head.

Slowly lift your torso, start walking in toward your head, raising your knees. There will come a point of balance where your toes will naturally lift off the floor.

Lift the toes, folding the feet so that they come close to the buttocks.

The steps leading to this point should be practiced for a number of days until you can do it slowly and fluidly.

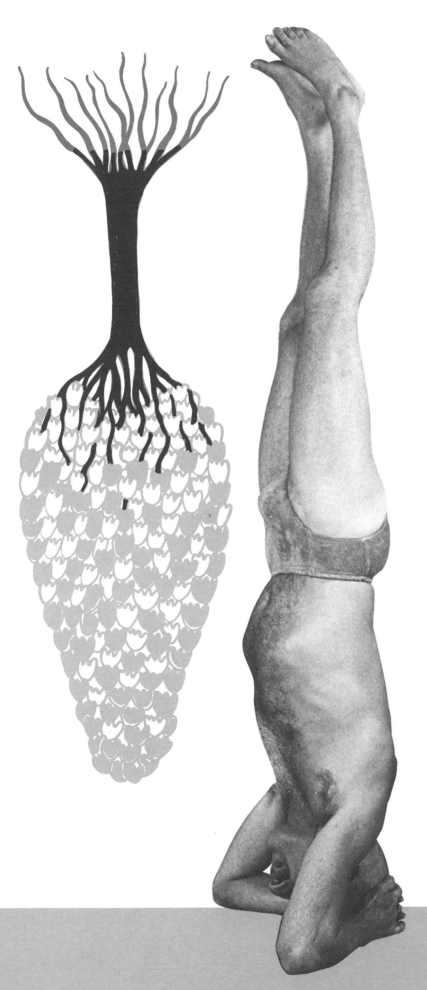

The Head Stand *Sirshasana*

From the Preliminary Head Stand posture, lift the thighs until they are parallel to the floor. Slowly straighten your legs in the air. The body should be all in a line. The weight is distributed between your elbows, head and hands. Hold for ten seconds and slowly reverse the positions, coming down to the floor again. There should be no jerking going into or coming out of the pose.

After coming down, rest for a minute in the Devotional pose, but with your hands spread in front of you. Then curve your head up to relieve any pressures in the neck. This rest gives the system a chance to readjust itself.

The Head Stand is an advanced pose and should be approached carefully. When it is mastered, it can be held for five minutes.

It is a pose that came into yoga history rather late. There have been elaborate claims made for it. Like the Shoulder Stand, there is a strong reverse flow of blood in the body; the brain receives a rich supply of blood as does the entire endocrine system.

The upper parts of the vertebrae are pressured while the lower part is relieved. This reversal helps bring flexibility into the lower part while building strength into the upper part.

If you feel sneezing or coughing coming on while in the posture, come down from it. Breathe through your nose in the posture. If you feel nauseous, or feel too much pressure, come down from the pose. Be sensitive to the body in the Head Stand and gauge its endurance accordingly. Smokers, drinkers and people with high blood pressure or sinus trouble should not do this posture.

The reverse sensation of the body in the air is very fluid and light, both physically and psychically. Everything is reversed, like the image of the tree. The sensation is of weightlessness, of walking in the air.

The image of the inverted tree is used in certain Hindu writings as a metaphor to illustrate that man, rather than being rooted on earth, has his highest energies flowing in from forces in the cosmos around him, infinite forces, still dimly understood.

80

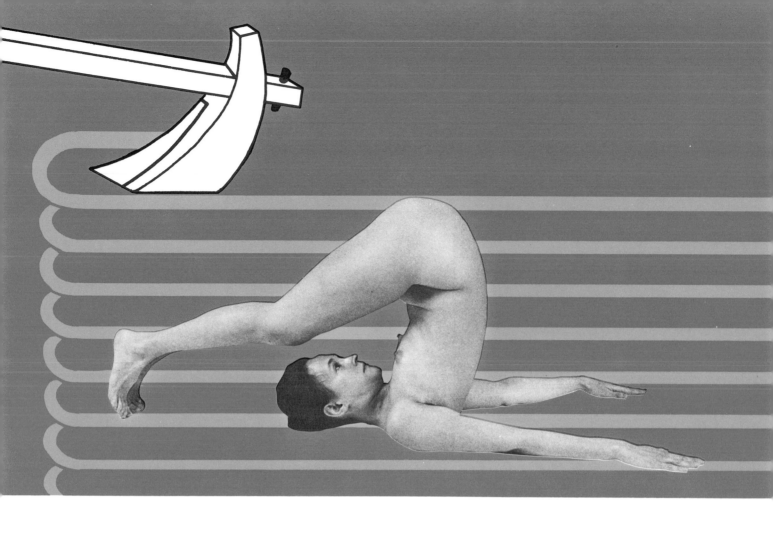

The Plow *Halasana*

From a supine position, move the legs up and over the head as in the Parallel Floor posture, and then proceed to slowly bend the torso even more, so that the toes touch the floor above your head. Keep your legs straight. Hold for as long as feels comfortable, breathing lightly. Now bring your feet up and slowly down to the floor.

The Spread Plow

From the Plow posture, slowly spread your legs as far apart as is comfortable. Bring your hands around and grab hold of your feet. Hold. Release and slowly return to a supine position.

The Plow is one of the best asanas for keeping the back flexible and stretching the muscles of the legs.

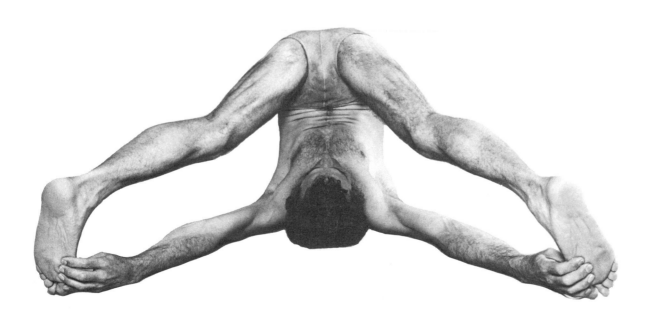

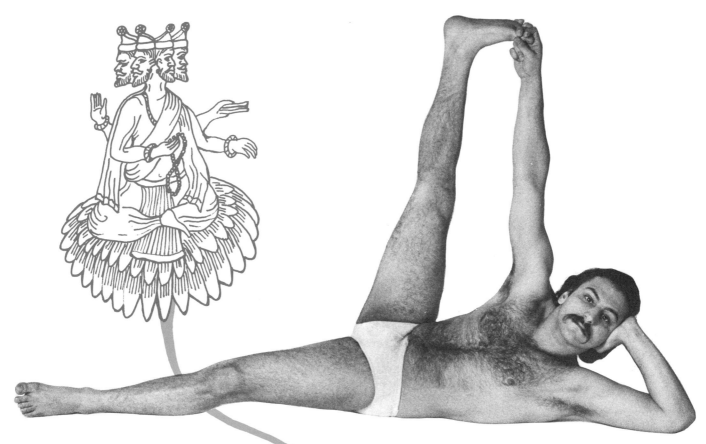

Vishnu's Couch

Lie on your side in a straight line. Your left arm is bent at the elbow and the hand cushions your head. Bend the right leg and grab the right big toe with your right hand. Slowly straighten the right leg so that it is at right angles to the body, still holding the toe. Lower the leg. Repeat and then do the other side.

In the primeval sea, Vishnu sleeps. He lies on a couch of the thousand-headed snake in the first position of the asana, a posture suggesting a lordly, controlled and dignified way of rest.

In his sleep a lotus grows from his navel, and from the lotus comes Brahman, the creative force who will shape the world and waken Vishnu, who then moves to the heavens. And so the creative umbilical circuit moves in two ways, giving birth and, in turn, awakening.

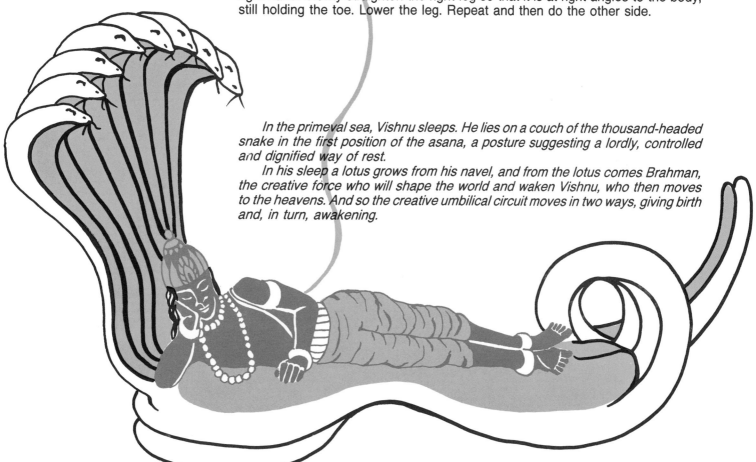

THE SUN

Many people in India, still conscious of man's dependence on nature, perform daily rituals to acknowledge their respect. The earth or floor at temples and holy places is walked on only with bare feet. Rivers are considered holy; daily bathing in them is conducted like a water rite. Ritual fires continually burn in many temples.

The sun, supreme fire element, is hailed as both the physical and spiritual center of all life; there are many temples devoted to its worship. In yoga, one pays tribute to the manifold powers of the sun by doing the following twelve-part asana. In one form of the exercise, twelve beneficent qualities of the sun are chanted, one for each movement.

This asana combines so many of the movements of the lying, crouching, stretching and standing postures that it is like a complete yoga routine; in fact, some teachers say that if you do twenty rounds, you have done your yoga for the day.

The ideal time to do this asana is at dawn, just when the sun is over the horizon.

"Face the sun, let its warm vibration raise the vibration of your body."

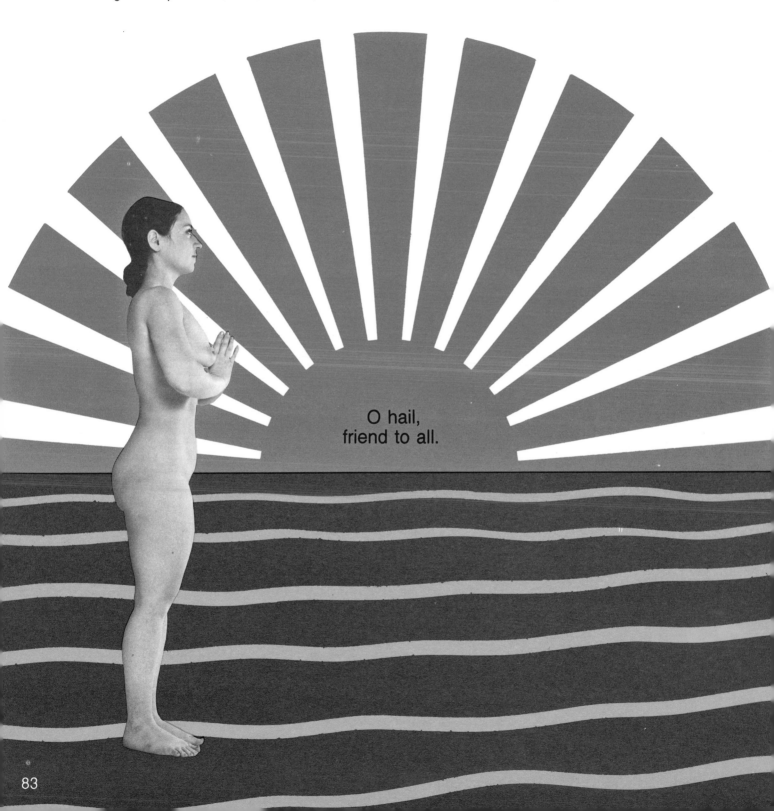

O hail,
friend to all.

83

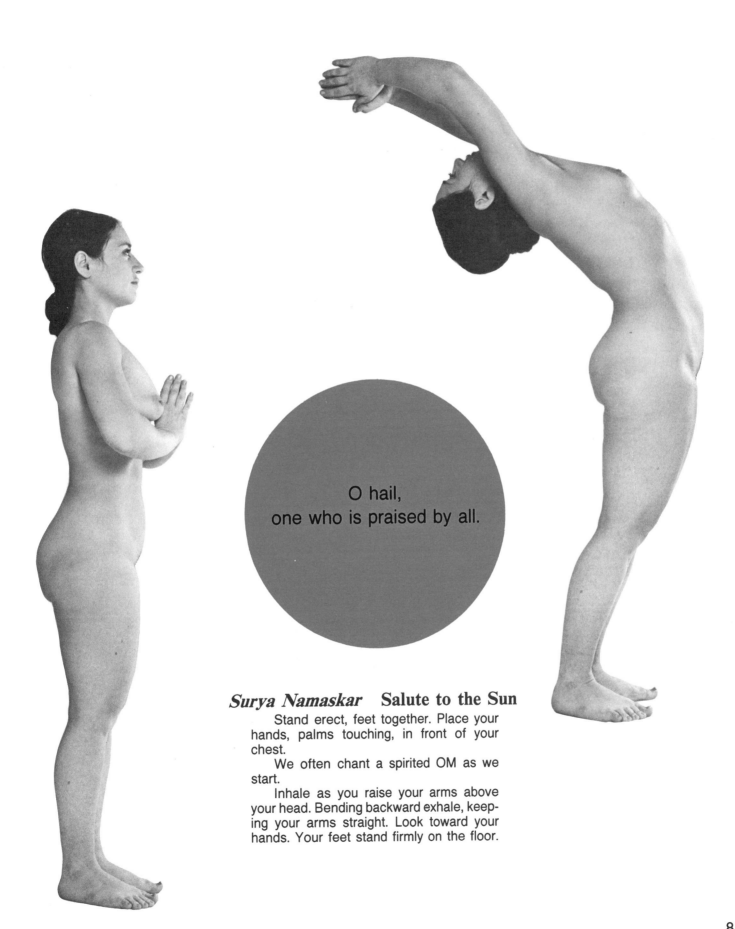

O hail,
one who is praised by all.

Surya Namaskar Salute to the Sun

Stand erect, feet together. Place your hands, palms touching, in front of your chest.

We often chant a spirited OM as we start.

Inhale as you raise your arms above your head. Bending backward exhale, keeping your arms straight. Look toward your hands. Your feet stand firmly on the floor.

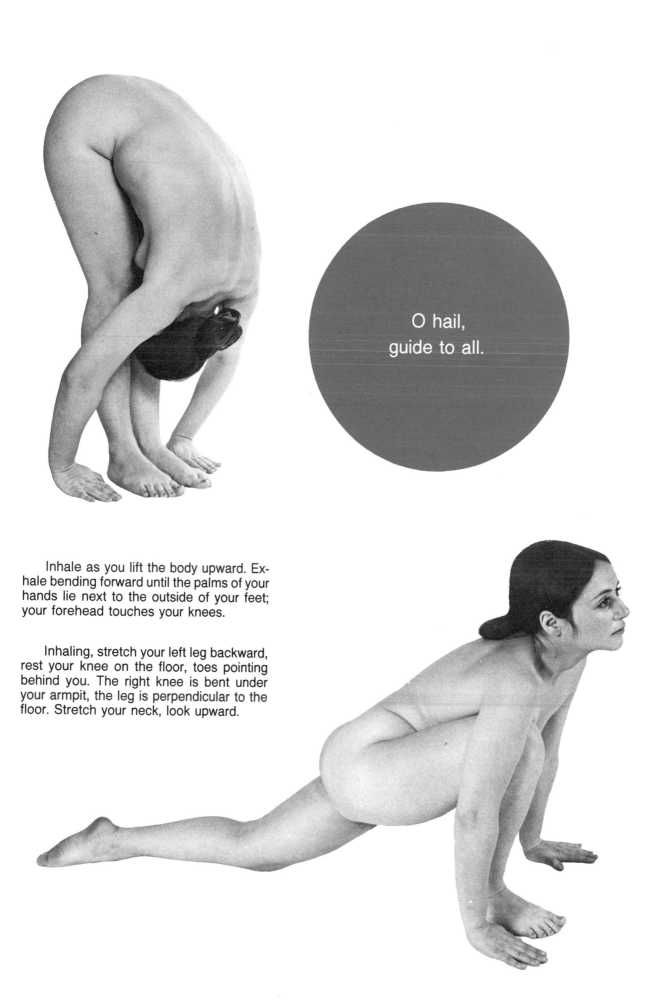

O hail,
guide to all.

Inhale as you lift the body upward. Exhale bending forward until the palms of your hands lie next to the outside of your feet; your forehead touches your knees.

Inhaling, stretch your left leg backward, rest your knee on the floor, toes pointing behind you. The right knee is bent under your armpit, the leg is perpendicular to the floor. Stretch your neck, look upward.

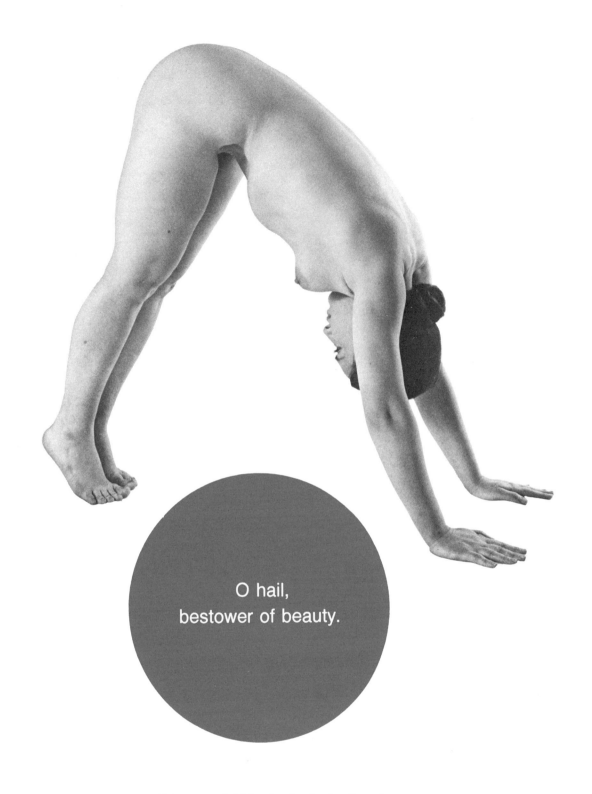

O hail,
bestower of beauty.

Bring your right leg back, placing it next to your left. Point your toes forward and exhale as you lift your buttocks, forming an arch with your body. Your head lies between your extended arms and faces toward your feet.

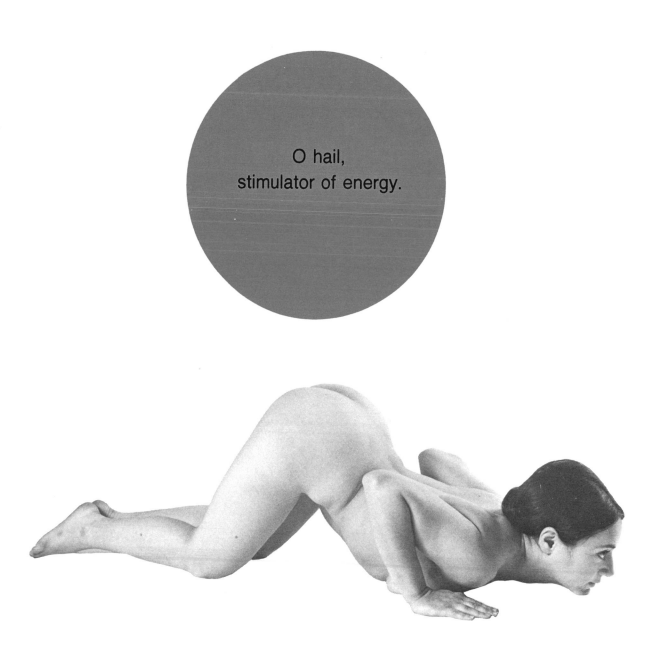

O hail,
stimulator of energy.

Inhaling, first bring your knees, then your chest, then your chin to the floor. The buttocks remain in the air. Your palms are flat on the floor along the outside of your chest.

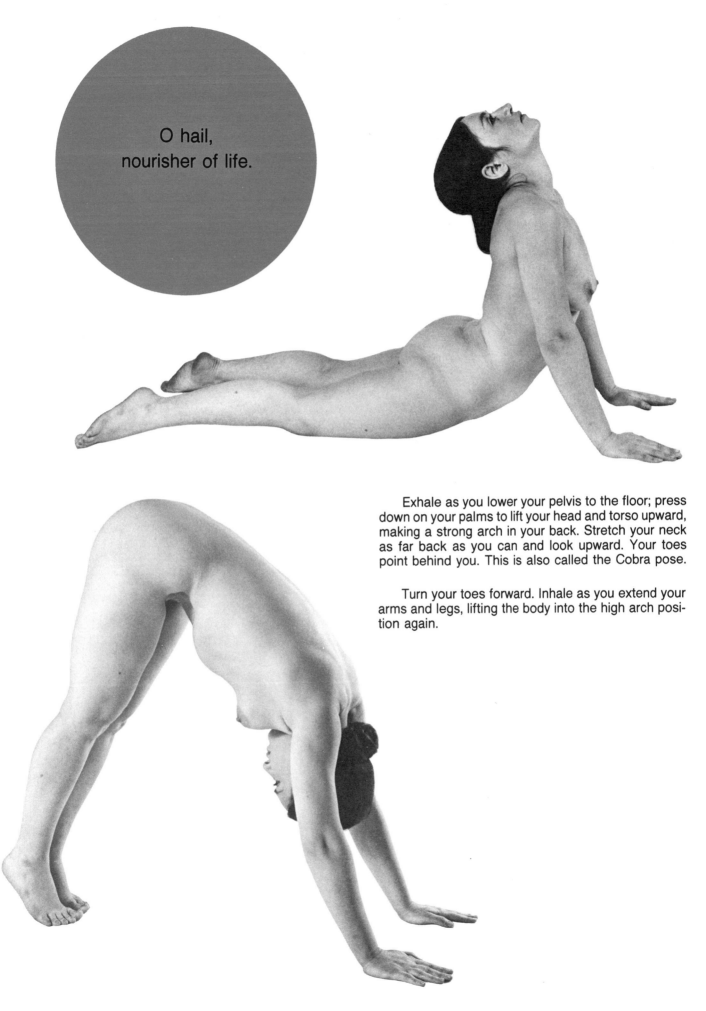

O hail,
nourisher of life.

Exhale as you lower your pelvis to the floor; press down on your palms to lift your head and torso upward, making a strong arch in your back. Stretch your neck as far back as you can and look upward. Your toes point behind you. This is also called the Cobra pose.

Turn your toes forward. Inhale as you extend your arms and legs, lifting the body into the high arch position again.

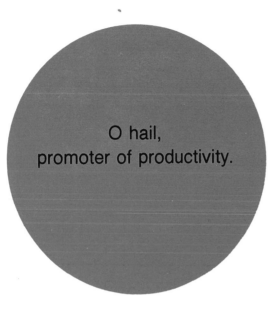

O hail,
promoter of productivity.

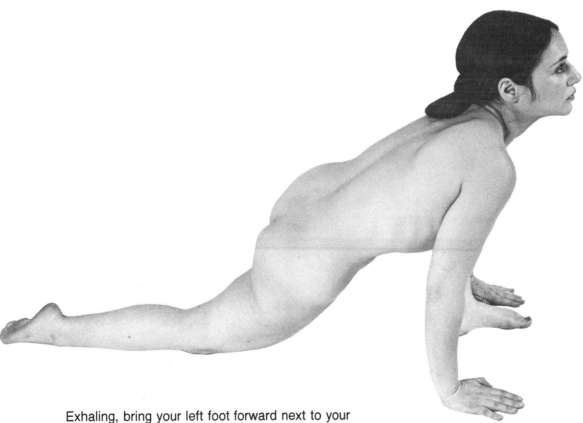

Exhaling, bring your left foot forward next to your left hand. The knee is bent under the armpit and the leg is perpendicular to the floor. Your right leg extends back, knee touching the floor, toes pointing backward. Look up.

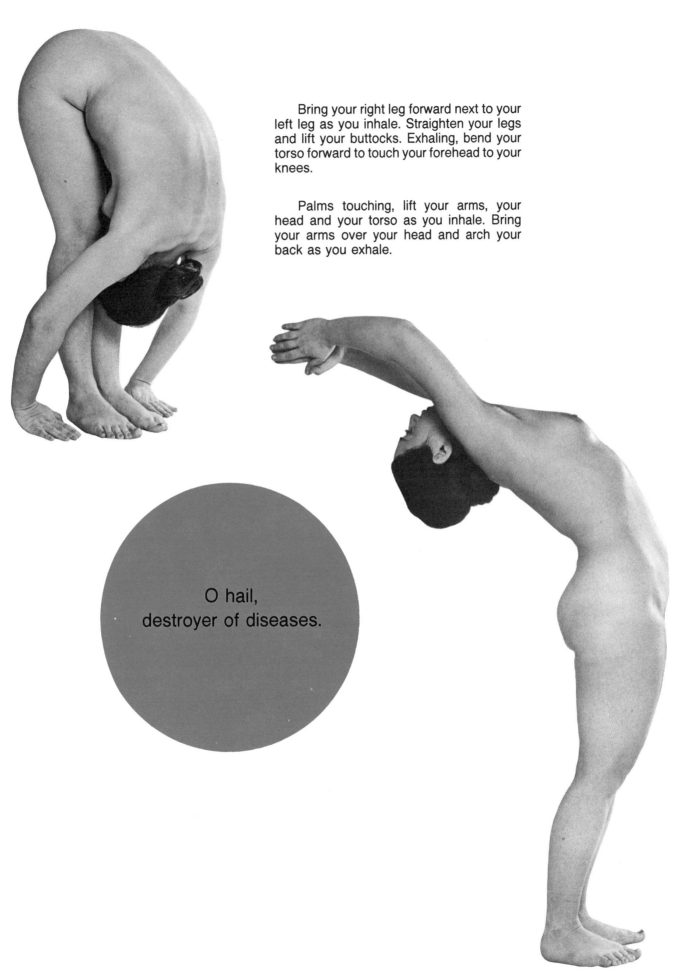

Bring your right leg forward next to your left leg as you inhale. Straighten your legs and lift your buttocks. Exhaling, bend your torso forward to touch your forehead to your knees.

Palms touching, lift your arms, your head and your torso as you inhale. Bring your arms over your head and arch your back as you exhale.

O hail,
destroyer of diseases.

90

O hail,
inspirer of awe.

O hail,
infuser of love.

O hail,
begetter of life.

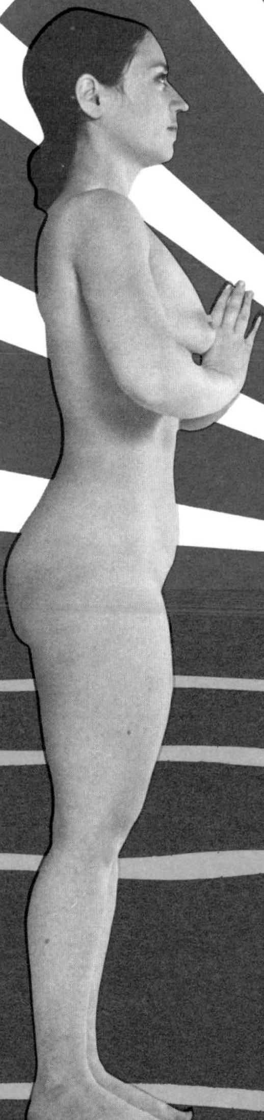

*May these twelve beneficent
qualities of the sun
befriend you
praise you
guide you
give you beauty
energy
nourishment
make you productive
healthy
loving
grace you with life
inspiration
effulgence.*

O hail,
effulgent one.

Inhale as you raise your arms and torso to stand erect. Bring your hands, palms together, to the front of your chest.

You have now completed 1 round of the Salute to the Sun. Practice at least 2 more rounds.

91

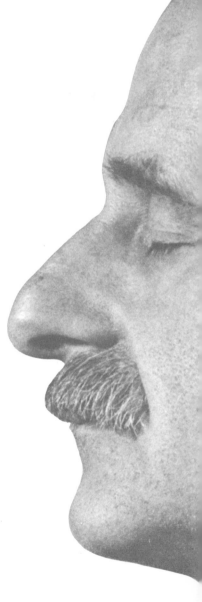

Pranayama
Advanced Breath Rhythms

Most of the nourishing energy for the body comes from the air we breathe and not, as commonly thought, from food or water. The control and regulation of the breath through Pranayama and breathing rhythms will bring increased nourishment to the body. In an earlier section of the book, we have learned how to open the lungs and coordinate the exercises with rhythmic breathing patterns. In this section we will deal with pranayama as a purifier, regulator and arouser of energy in the body.

The following two exercises use a mudra to facilitate the opening and closing of the nostrils. This particular hand gesture, illustrated on the next page, is called Vishnu mudra because the hand is held in the form of one of the symbols of the god Vishnu. Every religious member of the Vishnu sect paints this symbol on his forehead before he goes to temple in the morning. The large "U" shape stands for the female energy of the goddess–woman; the red teardrop form symbolizes the male.

To do Vishnu mudra place your right arm directly in front of your chest, elbow pointing straight down. The middle finger of your right hand rests on the bridge of your nose, the second and fourth fingers are curved next to your nostrils. The thumb and little finger are spread wide apart, the thumb representing the positive current of energy in the body and the little finger representing the negative current of energy.

In all of the following breathing exercises be sure to sit with your spine straight. You may use any of the sitting positions illustrated on page 10.

The Nerve Cleanser *Nadi Shoddhana*

In this exercise the breath is inhaled through the right nostril and exhaled through the left nostril in increasingly rapid succession.

Using Vishnu mudra, close the left nostril with your fourth finger as you breathe into your right nostril for a count of 6. Release the fourth finger and exhale through your left nostril for a count of 6 while closing the right nostril with your second finger. Repeat.

The sequence is: Inhale 6 Exhale 6 for two rounds
Inhale 4 Exhale 4 for two rounds
Inhale 2 Exhale 2 for two rounds

Now breathe in and out through alternate nostrils as rapidly as possible using the fingers to control the flow of air.

The Nerve Purifier *Nadi Shuddhi*

This alternate nostril breath is done in the same 2-to-1 ratio as the Rhythmic Breath (page 33).

With your hand placed in Vishnu mudra, close the left nostril with the fourth finger and slowly draw the air into the right nostril for the count of 4. With the second and fourth fingers close both nostrils and hold in the breath for the count of 2. Lift your fourth finger and slowly let out the breath from your left nostril for the count of 4. Close both nostrils and hold in the breath for the count of 2. Repeat.

The sequence is:
Inhale 4, hold in 2, exhale 4, hold out 2, for 2 rounds. When you feel comfortable with the hand position and breath count, increase the count.
Inhale 6, hold in 3, exhale 6, hold out 3, for 2 rounds. With daily practice you will slowly be able to increase the ratio to 20 to 10. Remember to proceed slowly and with a great deal of control so that you will not feel any strain.

By this measured and balanced rhythm of taking in, holding, releasing and holding out the air, you are setting up a cycle which is vivifying to the nervous and circulatory systems, a kind of internal massage.

Both of these pranayamas will make you feel light and energized. The mind will feel more alert and you will have better sleep and appetite.

Caste marks of different sects.

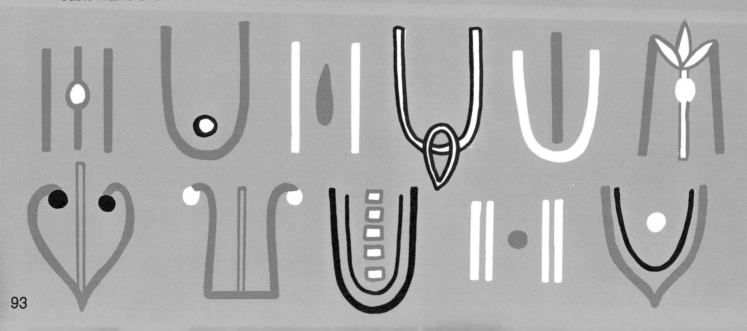

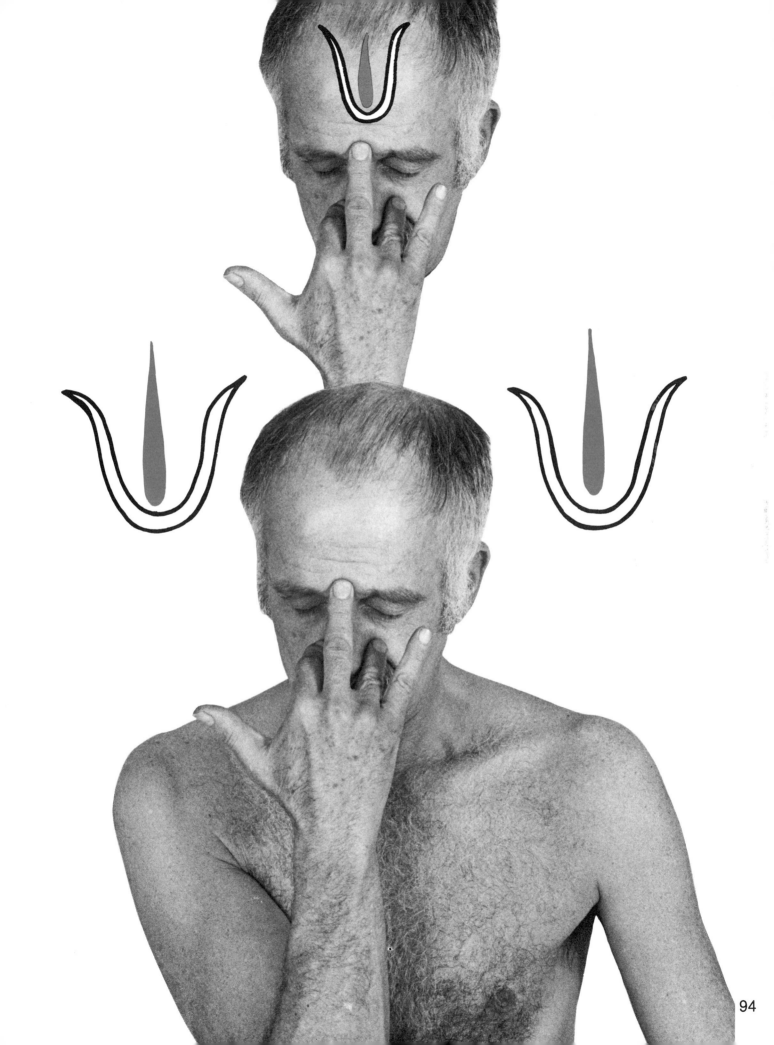

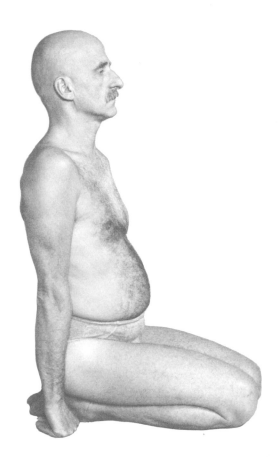

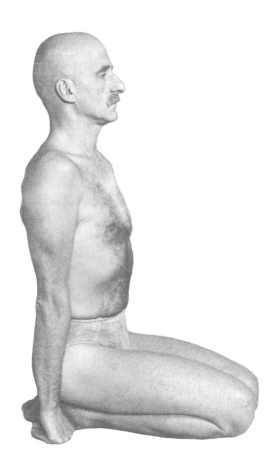

The Bellows Breath

As the air of a bellows fans a fire into activity, so the Bellows Breath arouses the body energy by bringing more oxygen into the blood stream. This classical pranayama gives the body more energy, endurance and stronger lungs.

When you are first learning this breathing exercise, it is best to sit in the Thunderbolt posture (page 11). This will enable you to check the movement of your diaphragm.

Sitting in the Thunderbolt posture, relax any tension in your body, calm your mind and concentrate your thoughts on the breath. Place your hand on the upper part of your diaphragm; now breathe deeply and feel your stomach move outward as you breathe in. Pull your stomach in as you breathe out. The inhalation and exhalation should be of equal duration.

When you feel comfortable directing the air to this part of your body, put your hand down by your side. Increase the speed and force of the breath so that you are moving the breath in and out in forceful, rapid succession. For the first week do only 20 rounds of this breath at a sitting. After each session relax the body by lying in any easy natural position. It is most important to allow the body to absorb the aroused energy before you go on to other activities.

When you feel at ease doing the 20 rounds, slowly increase the number of rounds each day until you reach the count of 60. If at any time you feel strain, stomach fibrillations or signs of tiredness, stop your practice for that day and relax. Resume the exercise the next day by doing fewer rounds.

After maintaining the level of 60 rounds for at least a week, again start to build the number of rounds until you reach the ideal count for this pranayama which is 120. You will be getting the optimum benefits of the exercise at this level, so it will be of no value to increase the count beyond this.

There is an enormous amount of energy flowing through the body when you have reached the 120 count. It is possible to contain and direct the energy by holding the breath for several seconds after the last round and channeling it through will power to the part of your body you feel needs vitalizing.

The Bee Breath

This breath is combined with sound. On the in-coming breath, the sound is like the low buzz of the male bee; on the out-going breath, it is like the high pitched hum of a female bee.

Sit in a comfortable position with your back straight. As you inhale slowly through your nose, make a low buzzing sound to vibrate the soft upper palate of your throat. Exhale very slowly bringing the vibration up into the nasal passages to make a high, humming sound. The exhalation should be twice as long as the inhalation. Keep your mouth closed while practicing several cycles of this breath.

The sound concentration causes the uvula to vibrate and secrete a fluid into the back of the throat. The sensation at first might make you cough, but this fluid is a valuable aid in creating a strong and harmonious voice. This breath also helps to rejuvenate the skin and clear up mucous conditions.

The Skull Shiner

In Hindi, the name for this pranayama, *Kapalabhati,* actually means to shine or brighten the skull. It is one of the classic cleansing techniques used in Hatha Yoga. The action of the breath in this exercise vibrates the tissues in the head which helps to drain the sinuses, cleanse the cerebrospinal fluids, relieve congestion in the skull cavity and also promote clearer thinking.

Sit in a comfortable position with your back straight. Slowly inhale deeply, now exhale deeply, eliminating as much air from the lungs as possible. Pull your stomach up under your rib cage and hold it there during the exercise. Now breathe in and out through the nose in short, quick breaths, just as you did in the Bellows Breath. The action this time, however, is in the top part of the chest. With daily practice, slowly increase the number of rounds of breath. When you reach the count of 40, concentrate the energy of the breath in a circular motion, moving from front to back, around the inside of the skull. It may take you several months of continual practice to reach the final count of 120 rounds. It is slow, steady progress that leads to true breath control.

Be sure to lie down and relax after each practice session.

People who have severe eye or ear disorders should not do this pranayama.

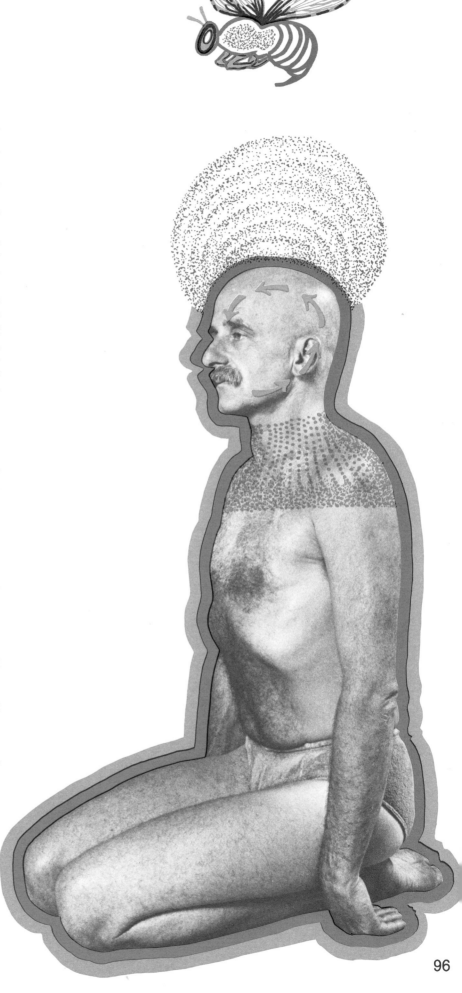

RELAXATION,

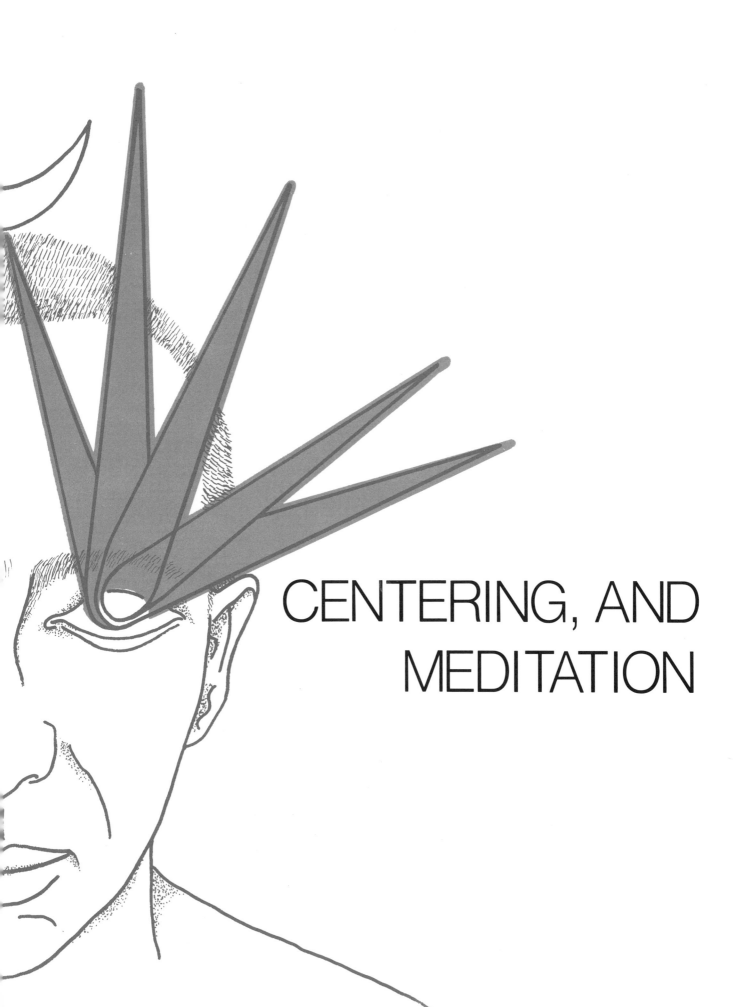

CENTERING, AND
MEDITATION

A relaxation after your daily yoga practice session will help quiet the body and contain the energies you have aroused. This should be an important part of your routine. If you don't relax for at least ten minutes after a full session you will feel hyperactive.

As you build a more healthful body with Hatha Yoga, you will have a new feeling for the body's internal and external rhythms, a sense of its wonder and dignity. This can begin to open one's whole awareness to a new kind of consciousness, and the centering exercises which follow will allow you to explore this area.

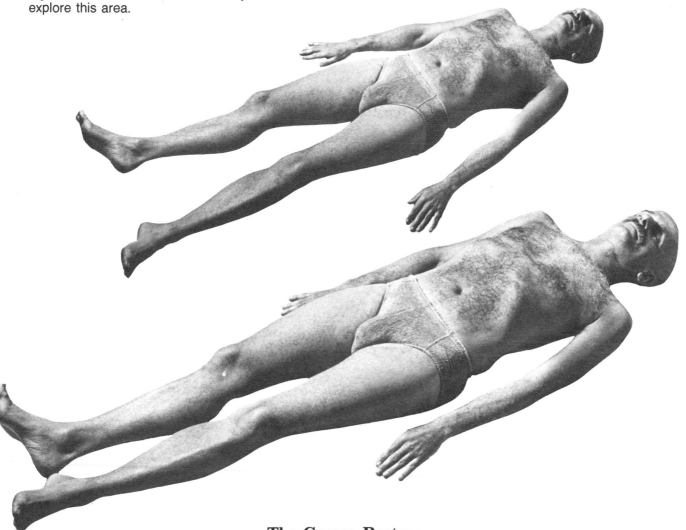

The Corpse Posture

Lie with your back on the floor. Your hands are relaxed at your sides, your feet stretched out in front of you, heels touching, toes spread apart.

In a variation, the feet and hands may be slightly spread open for a more casual position.

The Corpse posture itself can be used as a simple relaxation. By tensing the muscles, press your head, shoulders, back, pelvis, buttocks, thighs, calves and heels into the floor so that your body is as flat as possible; now relax. Repeat the tensing of the muscles, then lie in the relaxed position for several minutes.

This posture is excellent for relaxation and short naps and is used for the more complex techniques which will follow.

In this posture the body is in a balanced, structured form which allows it to relax while the mind is in a centered state of awareness. The aim of many of the meditations and concentrations is this state.

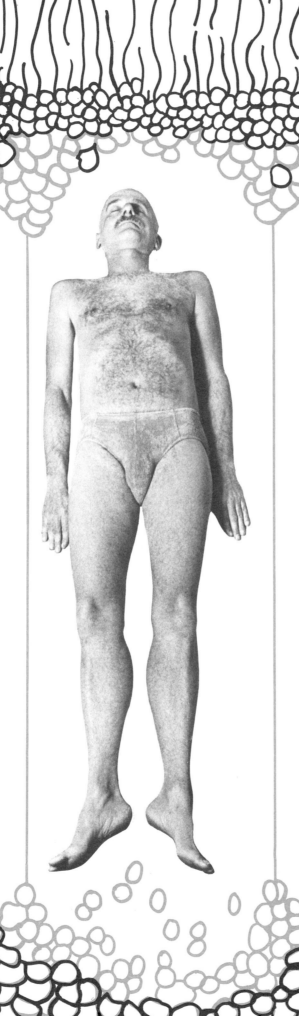

The Hollow Tube

Lie in the Corpse posture, hands at your sides. Imagine your body as a hollow tube with openings at the head and feet.

Imagine some gritty material like sand, soil, pebbles, or refuse like tar, sticks and underbrush, sludgy water, slag and even garbage.

Imagine any one of these materials rushing through the tube, starting at the opening at the top of the head and coming out the bottom of your feet. Visualize this continuous flow of impure material moving through you, by its very abrasiveness or weight causing a cleaning sensation in the body. Concentrate on this material running through your body until you feel a sensation of clean air or clear water flowing through the body. The tube that is the body becomes shining and clear, perhaps even transparent.

When the exercises in this section are successful for you, the transmitted thought forms open the creative–imaginative mind to make an intense visualization of the suggested process, which in turn causes certain sensations and movements in the physical body. The greater the concentration, the more intense the visceral effects.

This will be confirmed by certain experiences you may have, such as sweating in areas where heat is directed or tingling sensations where energies have been channeled.

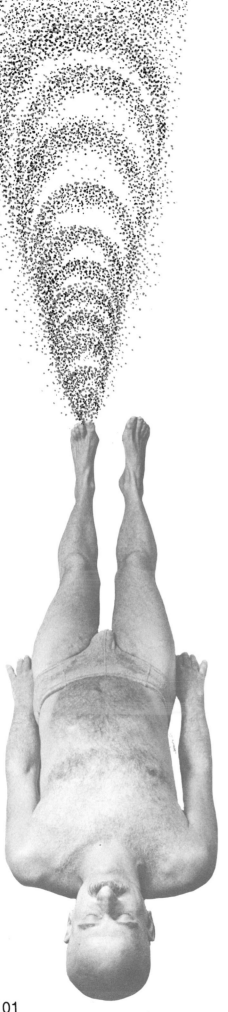

The Big Toe Energy Flow

Lie on the floor in the Corpse posture. Breathe deeply for at least 9 rounds. On the next inhalation concentrate on bringing all of your energy into the feet and then into your big toes.

Imagine your big toes growing with energy. Feel them expanding as they fill with a light, tingling sensation. First growing into the size of a lemon, then into the size of a grapefruit, the toes slowly getting larger and larger until they are as tall as you are. Feel them vibrating with glowing energy.

Now try to let this tingling vibration flow back into your feet; slowly move it through your ankles and into your calves. Inch by inch move this warm glow upward through your knees, thighs, crotch, pelvis, abdomen, diaphragm, chest and shoulders.

Concentrate on the fingertips until you feel this warming sensation.

Slowly let it climb through your arms and join the energy resting at your shoulders. Now move this energy through your neck, throat, chin, mouth, cheeks, ears, nose, eyes, forehead and back of your head to the crown of your skull. Your body should feel very light, even floating, the top of your head glowing. A feeling of relaxation pervades.

Energy Spiral *Yoga Nidra*

Lie in the Corpse posture. Extend your arms to your sides at shoulder level. Breathe in for 8 counts, hold your breath for 4 counts, exhale 8 counts and hold out the breath for 4 counts. Do at least 9 rounds of this rhythmic breath.

On the tenth round think of positive energy entering the top of your head as you breathe in, traveling through your head, neck, shoulders, chest and diaphragm to your navel like a wave of light or heat. Hold this energy at the navel while you hold the breath. As you exhale think of negative energy entering your feet, perhaps in the form of a cool breeze, traveling up through your legs, thighs, crotch and pelvis and resting at the navel while you hold out the breath.

Relax your concentration on the breath, and bring all of your attention to the energies centered at your navel.

Feel a pulse beat of energy at your navel. You are going to visualize this dot of energy slowly spiraling outward until it encircles your body. Start at the very center of your navel, feel a line of energy circling outward very, very slowly; first the size of a dime, it grows larger to the size of a quarter making concentric circles clockwise around the navel, growing slowly larger and larger until your body is contained within a circle of energy. The circle lies about six inches above your head and below your feet.

Imagine yourself within a glowing orb of golden light. Let this radiance fill your body for a few minutes. Then start to spiral the circle of energy inward, making counterclockwise circles, very slowly following along the same path of direction as you move in toward the navel. Screw the line of energy tightly into the navel. This concentration will lead you into a deep state of relaxation. You will feel as though your body has fallen asleep, but your mind will be alert and aware of everything around you. Allow at least twenty minutes to go through this whole process.

This exercise should be done under very quiet conditions. Any disturbance during this exercise may be shocking to the psyche. If you feel uneasy at any time while doing this concentration, stop and just open your eyes and become conscious of the room and your body lying on the floor.

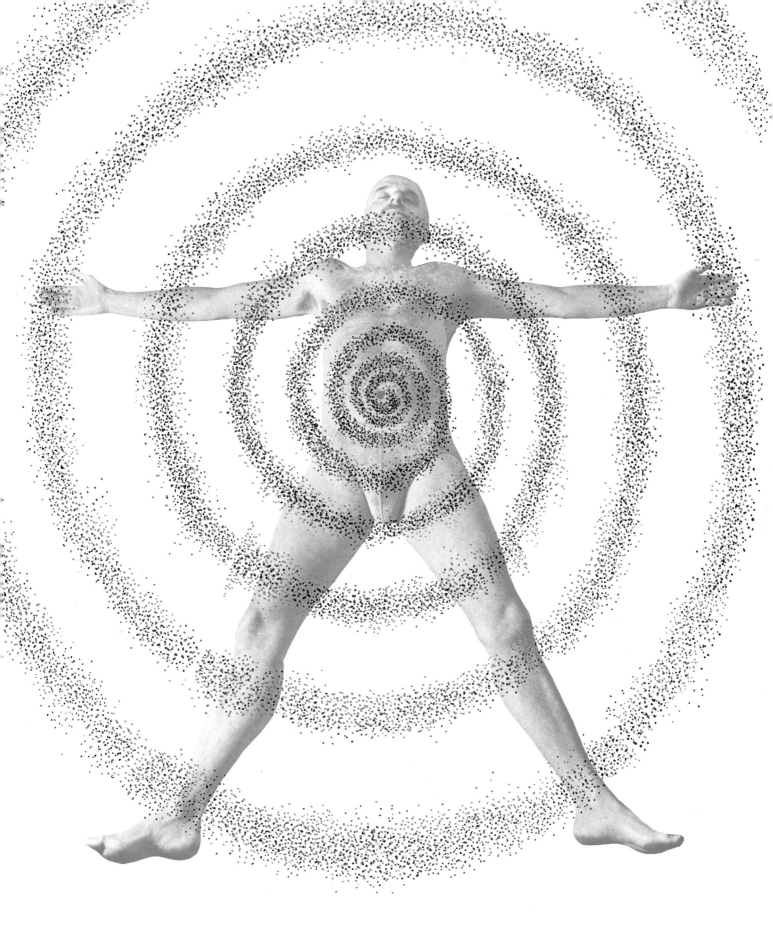

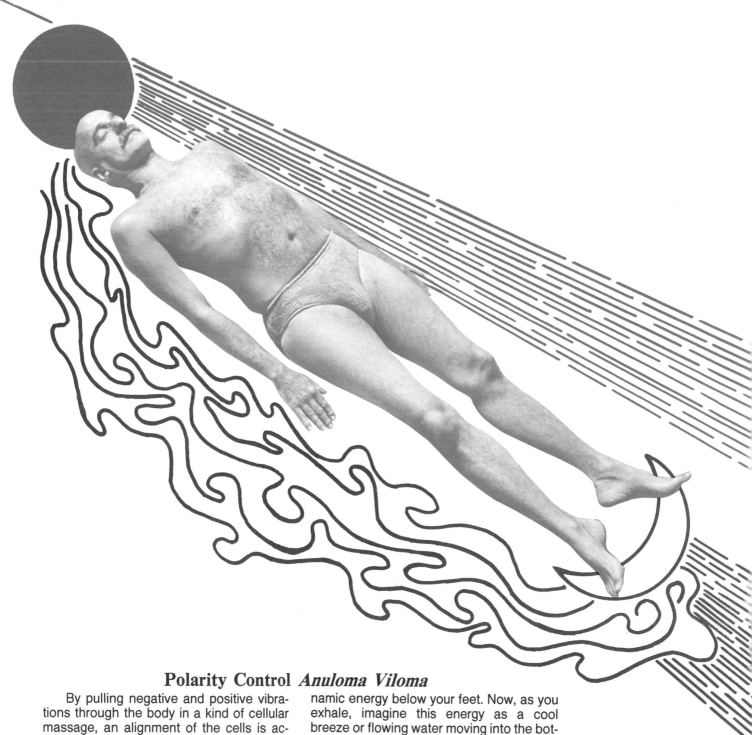

Polarity Control *Anuloma Viloma*

By pulling negative and positive vibrations through the body in a kind of cellular massage, an alignment of the cells is accomplished. Each cell has a polarity, magnetic in quality like the earth. A balanced polarity contributes to a balanced psyche and body.

Lie on the floor with your head to the north, your feet pointing toward the south. Do at least 9 rounds of Rhythmic Breathing (inhale 8, hold the breath 4, exhale 8, hold out the breath 4). Now close your eyes, imagine a large sunlike energy hovering over your head. As you breathe in, draw this sun energy in through the top of your head, slowly moving it inch by inch through the body. When you reach the bottom of your feet at the end of the inhalation, let the energy filter out through the soles of the feet.

Hold in the breath and think of cool dy-namic energy below your feet. Now, as you exhale, imagine this energy as a cool breeze or flowing water moving into the bottom of your feet and slowly flowing upward through the body until it comes out the top of the head.

Hold out the breath and again think of the sun energy above your head. Repeat, drawing these energies back and forth through the body, the sun energy on the in-breath, the cool breeze, negative energy, on the out-breath.

Do this exercise slowly and rhythmically until a light, floating feeling develops. Stop the concentration at this point and rest in this deep state of relaxation. Your breathing will become very light; it may even stop for a short while. Don't worry—breathing is an involuntary reflex, so when your body needs oxygen again, you will inhale.

103

Emotion Release

In the last few exercises we have been centering and relaxing the body; next we will try to deal with one of the links between body and mind—the emotions.

Often when we feel tension and tightness in the body it is caused by our holding on to a feeling that we haven't been able to express. There are anger, joy, sadness, hurt and ecstasy all locked into areas of our body.

Sometimes one can be aware of a specific hurtful experience that causes a part of the body to become tense. For instance, a feeling of heaviness in the head or chest may develop just after a strong argument. At other times the tension is more subtle and difficult to trace.

Lie in the Corpse posture. Do some deep, easy breathing to relax the body. Slowly, starting with the toes, go through the body trying to find some kind of feeling like tension or an ache, a twitch or even a tingle. By concentrating on the area this feeling is coming from, images of emotions may spontaneously arise. For example, one student, while concentrating, felt a great pressure on his ears and immediately remembered a time of near drowning in the ocean. He hadn't realized the anxiety of that earlier experience was still with him.

If emotions arise, try to reexperience them deeply. Release them by opening your eyes, by sensing present time intensely as a cleanser to the past.

Do this exercise in a private place where you will not be afraid to show emotion. Remember you are in control of the exercise. If you feel shaky from the emotions, make them positive. That is one of the points of the exercise.

Love Release

The love concentration releases love–energy–feeling.

Sit in one of the Lotus postures, eyes closed. Still the mind, breathe lightly.

Think of yourself. Create a very positive image of yourself from all your positive qualities and actions. Feel good feelings for yourself, affectionate, complimentary and respectful.

Think of someone you love of the same sex, a near and dear friend. Think of all the really lovable things in that person. Feel how that love is given to you. Feel grateful and loving towards that person.

Think of someone you hardly know whom you may see often but perhaps don't even talk to. Think of that person with kindness and love. Wish him well.

Think of someone you hate someone you feel has really hurt you deeply in your life. Try to understand the makeup of that person. Feel compassion and then straight affection for that person. Imagine yourself embracing that person.

Envision yourself in a line with all the people you have just concentrated on. Send out feelings of love to each of them in turn and then to all of them together. Expand your feeling of lovingness toward them.

Now think of all the humans in this world. See them in all their struggles and pleasures, their kindnesses and loving efforts. Send all the love that has been building.

Do each part of this concentration for five minutes.

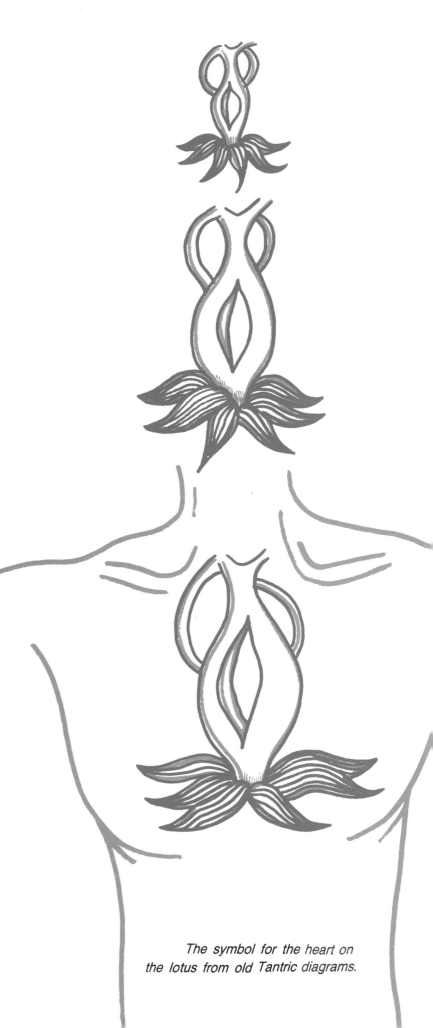

The symbol for the heart on the lotus from old Tantric diagrams.

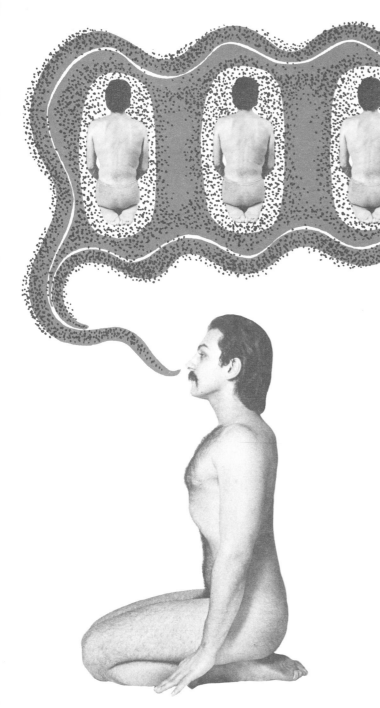

Following the Breath

There are many different systems of meditation, but most start with some form of inner concentration. These systems all lead to a remarkably similar point, to the yoga, the union.

Various structures have been charted and passed down to us by men who have had remarkably deep and powerful meditative experiences.

We present some of these meditations as beginning seed stages from which your own discipline can grow.

To some, they will lead to further investigations into reading meditative writings. For others, the practice may clarify the need for further concentration with a teacher.

It is for you to find ways of meditation that reveal something to you, that can open the adventure of the inner life.

May the lotus flower
And all other flowers
Kind flowers
Blossoming flowers
Silky flowers
Strange flowers
Fragrant flowers
Subtle flowers
Open, open for you.

Sit in the Thunderbolt posture. (If this is difficult, sit in any comfortable sitting pose.) Have a clock at your side.

Breathe deeply in and out through the nose for 9 rounds. Watch the breath as it moves in and out of the lungs.

Now, before drawing in the breath, think the number 1, breathe in and exhale, then think the number 2. Continue counting before each round of inhalation and exhalation until you reach the number 10. Start again at 1, do this for five minutes.

For the second part, breathe in and out and then think the number, placing it *after* the round of breath. Count each round of breath until 10 and then start again at 1, for the next five minutes.

Now put your full concentration on the breath. Watch it closely, follow its movement in and out of the lungs for five minutes.

Continue breathing, concentrating now on the tip of your nose at that place where the air current moves in and out. Feel the sensation of the movement at this point. Hold the concentration at the tip of your nose for five minutes.

Now think of an image that characterizes the movement of the breath, a leaf in the breeze, a flag flying, a ripple on water, any image that comes naturally to you. Concentrate on that image. The breath proceeds on its own, more quietly and slowly. Do this for five minutes.

After this twenty-five minute period, lie down on the floor and relax or, if you still feel in the meditative mood, remain sitting and allow it to continue.

This exercise trains you for extreme concentration; it especially enables you to remove all other thoughts from your mind. You can do this meditation every day. Watch it closely. It will start to teach you.

Be patient. Some days the concentration will be better than others.

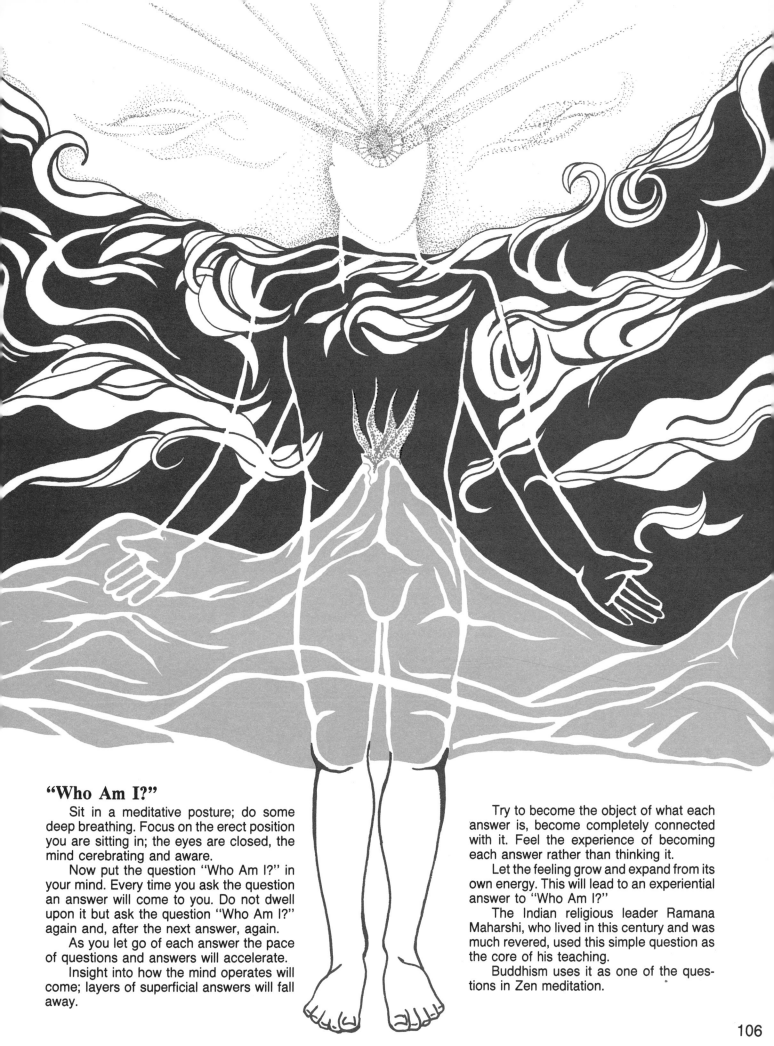

"Who Am I?"

Sit in a meditative posture; do some deep breathing. Focus on the erect position you are sitting in; the eyes are closed, the mind cerebrating and aware.

Now put the question "Who Am I?" in your mind. Every time you ask the question an answer will come to you. Do not dwell upon it but ask the question "Who Am I?" again and, after the next answer, again.

As you let go of each answer the pace of questions and answers will accelerate.

Insight into how the mind operates will come; layers of superficial answers will fall away.

Try to become the object of what each answer is, become completely connected with it. Feel the experience of becoming each answer rather than thinking it.

Let the feeling grow and expand from its own energy. This will lead to an experiential answer to "Who Am I?"

The Indian religious leader Ramana Maharshi, who lived in this century and was much revered, used this simple question as the core of his teaching.

Buddhism uses it as one of the questions in Zen meditation.

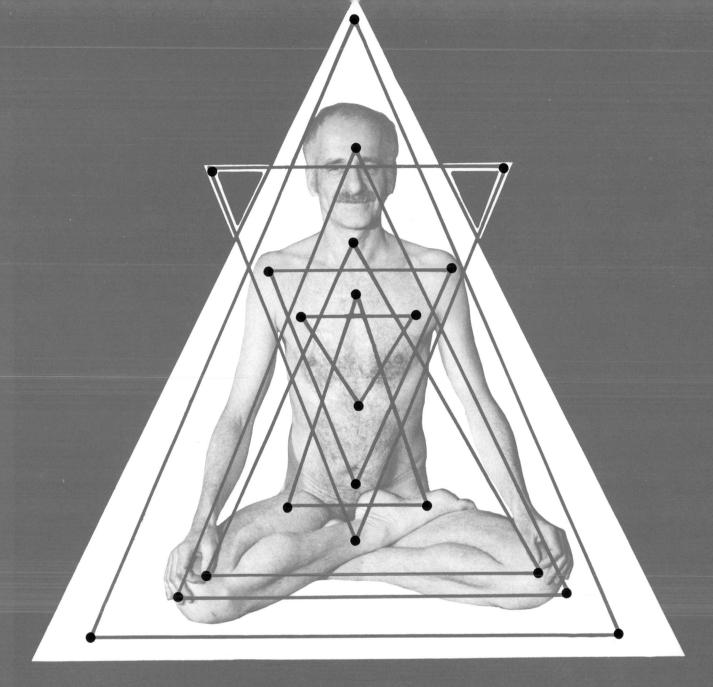

Body Triangles

This series of exercises will make you aware of certain energy points, or *bindus,* in the body. Many are located at nerve vortices. Through them energies of a higher vibrational nature can be drawn into the body.

They are used in meditative practice as points of concentration and for the gathering and movement of energy forces. Other cosmic points exist as extended force lines outside the body and can be used in the concentration as linkages to those within the body.

Through simple inner concentration, they can often be seen or felt within us as small glowing orbs, as geometric forms, or as forms within forms.

The triangular forms (in the diagram) all extend from a line of connected points starting at the base of the spine and ascending to a point that seems to hover just above the cranium.

• Close your eyes. Concentrate on finding the placement of each of the body bindus. Refer to the diagram; each blue dot is a bindu. Hold the concentration on each one for about a half minute.

• Concentrate on the three bindu constituents of each triangle, and see if you can become aware of the energy lines flowing through them. These movements are stimulated by nerve currents.

• Sit in the Lotus position, and imagine the apex of a triangle starting at the top of the head, moving down the outside of the shoulders to points on the ground just below each knee, completing itself by the base line of the triangle moving along the ground below the body. Concentrate on the triangle; concentrate very hard on the triangle and try to forget the body. Imagine the triangle filled with pure glowing energy, your energies, creating a field within the triangle. Feel the triangle glow from the energy within it. Now try to draw energy into the triangle by taking a series of long deep breaths.

When the glow seems most intense, hold the breath as long as it is comfortable. Then exhale and breathe quietly.

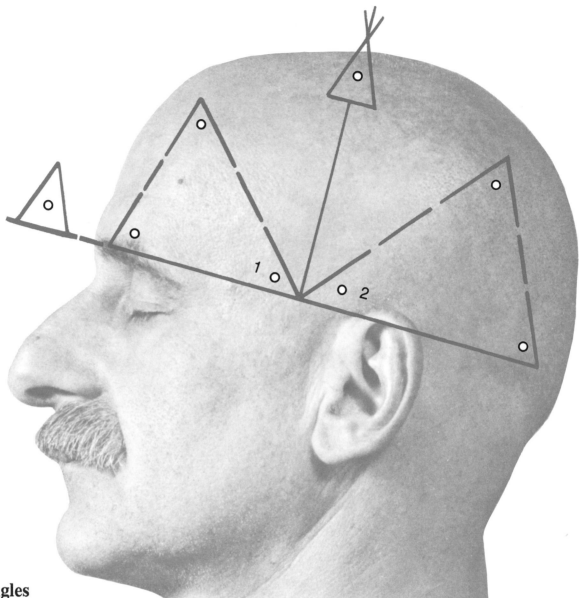

Head Triangles

A series of more refined bindus, energy points, are located in the head, some of their physical counterparts being the pituitary gland (bindu 1) and the pineal gland (bindu 2).

They are located at seven main points in the cranial area (as diagramed). The seven pranic rays, *suptapundum,* come into the head at these points. The experience of these flowing energies will sometimes occur in·meditation.

The three in the front and the three back points form themselves into triangles. In another grouping, the lower bindus fall into a line which starts at the point of the third eye and moves between the folds under the brain, sloping downward toward the back of the head.

As with the body bindus, they are used for concentration and the movement of pranic energy. By strong concentration, the points will become specific. As you work to find the bindus, the body will spontaneously help you to locate them.

• The following exercise will help you learn to move energy along the lower line of bindus in the head. Concentrate on the bindu at your third eye, a point

midway between your eyebrows.

Run an imaginary line, slanting downward, from this point to a point four inches behind it inside of the head (bindu 2). Concentrate on this second bindu until you feel the energy emanating from it.

Using the Rhythmic breath, breathe in for the count of 8 and feel the energy flowing outward along the line leading to the third eye. Move it through the third-eye bindu out to a point in space 4 inches directly in front of the head. Concentrate on this bindu while holding the breath for a count of 4, so that it becomes a specific point of energy. As you exhale to the count of 8, run the energy back along the same line through the third eye to bindu 2. Hold the energy there while holding the breath for 4 counts.

Repeat, drawing the energies out along this line, out of the head on the in-breath and into the head on the out-breath.

Practice of this exercise will increase and sharpen your powers of concentration and make you aware of different levels of consciousness.

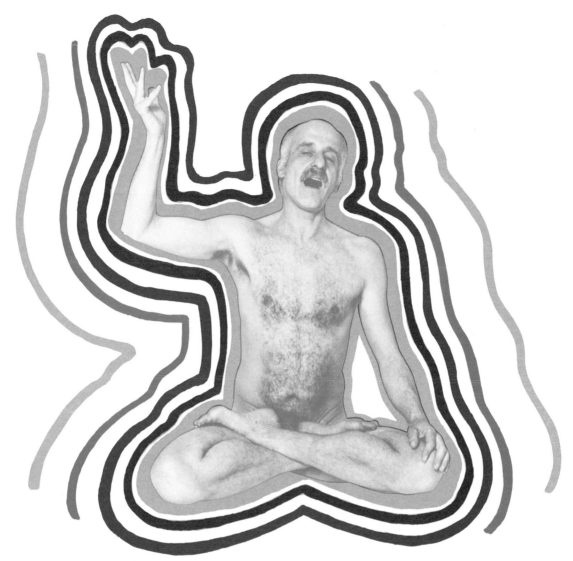

Sound as Meditation

Mantra is the yoga of vibrational sound. The stress is on the vibrational impact of the sound on the body and mind.

It is an ancient science, developed thousands of years ago in India, using sounds from the Sanskrit alphabet. It often deals with single-linked chanted sounds without word meanings.

Mantra became so highly developed that there exists a sound to vibrate and activate each part of the body. There are thousands of different kinds of mantras.

In India, the father privately gives his son a certain mantra as an initiation into maturity. The guru–teacher gives a personal mantra of initiation to the aspirant; certain mantras are the religious songs of the Indian people. Many mantras are simple phrases in benediction of the gods or the life force. The gods characterize different aspects of man's manifold nature, and the particular vibrational sound of his name has an interior effect, physical as well as psychological.

Mantra should be heard. Start to chant. Mantra is chanted out loud, mantra is chanted interiorly without the voice.

● Sit in any simple sitting position. Chant OM as we did in the earlier lung opening exercise (p 30). Now chant the OM only for itself. Feel its vibrational nature. Chant it as a slow, long, sustained sound. As the breath ends, quiet the vibration so that there is a gradual transition to the silence.

● Sit with a group of people in a circle. Hold hands and chant the OM together. You will discover its remarkable nature.

● Do a shorter continued repeated sound on the OM. This is called japa.

● Move back and forth between the long OM and the japa according to your feelings.

● Sit with a group. Sing the OM freely. Sense your own rhythms and the rhythms of the group. Meld them together.

● Look at an object, any object. Try to feel its vibration. Make a sound that seems to express the object. Repeat the sound. Try to merge with the object through the sound.

● Sit in a group. Let each person chant any sound or series of sounds that they feel. Let the orchestration grow naturally. Feel open-ended about how long the chanting should go on, even if it be hours. In a more controlled way the Hare Krishna group uses a continual mantra throughout the day as a form of worship.

● Take the longer HARE OM (pronounced hah ree aum), meaning praise the OM, the universal essence sound. Use the two words as a structure. Vary it, raise it, lower it, speed it, laugh it, cry it. Feel it, feel its vibration, feel its meaning. After a while, it will sing itself.

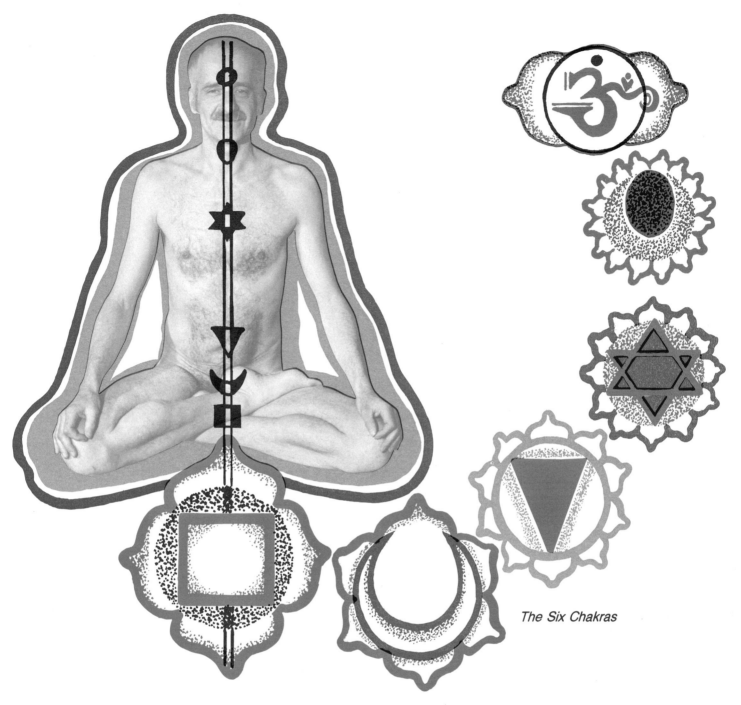

The Six Chakras

Mandala, Color and Shape for Meditation

Mandalas, in simple and complex forms, are centering mechanisms. They are diagrams of colors and shapes, often used in conjunction with sound. They are used in most cultures as part of spiritual and healing practice.

Through visual stimulus they effect the psyche in the same way as the meditations and mantras. Instead of requiring inner visualization, forms are presented in which one's eyes follow along the surface of the mandala and are taken into the mind and psyche for inner visualization.

Gods, goddesses, animals, plants and other symbols all have particular meanings for the meditator, arousing certain emotions and states of consciousness, so that one's involvement becomes a dynamic set of changing experiences all aimed at an ultimate mind centering.

Most modern Western versions of mandalas tend merely to bombard or spiral the mind or to be decorative.

The outer form of the mandala is often circular, mirroring circling energy patterns in the body. If square, it is often similar in each quadrant, the quadrant drawn in such a way as to face inward like petals of a flower.

The inner meditation forms, or *yantras,* are often geometric in nature too, reflecting energy patterns in the mind and body, an archetypal mathematics found in all nature.

In the really complex geometrics the mind is forced to follow very careful steps of concentration. Sustained energy and refined skill in holding the mind are required. In the Shri Yantra every small triangle and the larger triangles that have created them are concentrated upon, and in the meditation each one has a specific meaning.

110

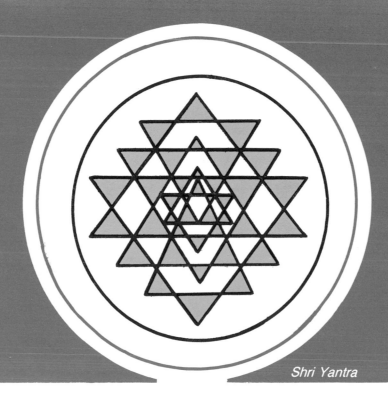

Shri Yantra

Central to certain areas of yoga is the study of the chakras, mandalas which represent a series of spinning psychic energy centers at points along the spinal column. Each chakra has a specific color, significant because it illustrates the vibrational level of consciousness that emanates from that center.

The different shapes in the chakras were each developed to be used for inner visualization (at the places in the body diagramed on the previous page) to activate respective areas in the body.

A yellow square at the base of the spine, a silver crescent moon slightly higher, an inverted red triangle at the navel, a six-pointed blue star in the area of the heart, a fuchsia oval around the throat and an orange or black dot at the point of the third eye are concentrated upon, each in turn.

The point of this action is to raise the latent energy at the base of the spine through each center to the crown of the head in order to attain an experience of the superconscious mind. It is the Yoga of the Kundalini and is an involved practice using the sounds for each of the petals plus the seed sound shown as a Sanskrit letter in the middle of each chakra.

People with psychic abilities have been able to see the chakric colors as emanations from the body. These could be connected to auras that are also seen around the body and head. Scientists through Kirlian photography are starting to record these phenomena.

The real knowledge of Kundalini Yoga and chakra gazing should be studied with a teacher. However, as a beginner you can try to locate these centers of energy by yourself.

Gaze at a yellow square you have made for fifteen seconds. Close your eyes and try to visualize the square. Open your eyes and gaze again on the yellow square, this time for twenty seconds. Close your eyes and see if you can now visualize the square.

Repeat exterior and interior gazing upon the square until you can hold onto the image with your eyes closed. (It is possible that the color of the square may change in the inner visualization.) When you can clearly see the image for at least thirty seconds with your eyes closed, take a deep breath and bring the square down along the spinal column until it finds its proper place.

Do this same exercise for the yantric symbol in each chakra using a drawn silver crescent, inverted red triangle, blue star, fuchsia oval and black dot.

This is just one of the ways in which these symbols can be used, a kind of elementary exercise, but one that takes much concentration. The exercise can activate the physical area in the body to which it corresponds.

ENLIGHTENMENT	Samadhi, satori
CONTEMPLATION	Dyhana
CONCENTRATION	Dharana
GATHERING IN	Pratyahara

THE ROYAL PATH LEADING TO STILLING OF THE MIND   RAJ YOGA

All of the previous meditations have to do with the stilling of the mind. Stilling doesn't mean not using the mind. It means thinking from another plane, a clearer, more direct (and directed) place.

This plane of consciousness is called the super-conscious mind and the intuitive mind. In concentrated activity it is that mind we sometimes experience when creative ideas and solutions—in any area of our lives, whether simple or complex—seem just to flow without a strong exercise of will. This we often call inspiration.

When we are talking and find ourselves saying things of a perceptive nature, making unusual thought linkages, getting to the root of things, saying things we hadn't thought before, when the sensation is of the conscious mind seeming to listen to thoughts coming from an unknown level of awareness, this is the super-conscious mind at work.

It is the telepathic mind, the prophetic mind, the subtle mind, it is the place of elevated feeling.

One must experience and know its dimensions to be able really to use it. Our orientations in society, in education, in our work life and even in our religious life do not usually lead in this direction.

Hallucinogenic drugs have a place in the history of reaching this creative state of consciousness. However, trying to approach the superconscious state by the use of this outer stimulus has nothing to do with the way of yoga, which is intent on building lasting inner awareness and strength.

It is this mind that the Raj yogis try to contact, to strip into clarity, to be able to use at any moment. It is the mind without ego, in tune with the universe, the larger ego.

The few men and women who live in this nearly egoless state are the seers and the prophetic ones; they have the vision, and they embody the vision by the lives they lead. They are our spiritual teachers.

What they teach is that each of us can move upward on the ladder of consciousness. What they also teach is that ultimately we are our own teachers. When our awareness grows, we can learn from every occurrence and every person in our lives.

This yogic idea of transforming our spiritual–moral self is an expression of the same optimistic outlook which, on another level, we Westerners hold as the democratic ideal of the self-made man.

All the stages of spiritual growth are within known structures, available in literature. From these books one can come to know and understand them with the conscious mind, but for the real knowledge they must be experienced.

The gathering-in process, *pratyahara,* involves quieting all the senses. That is why one closes the eyes, breathes lightly and sits in a quiet place.

Through the various centerings in this book you have had the experience of "concentration," *dharana.* It is the process of concentration leading to single-pointed concentration. All other things are cleared from the mind.

In "contemplation," *dyhana,* having centered in on the object of concentration, a single intense image is held; the experience is no longer one of thought, but the thought and the thinker are one.

In the enlightenment stage, *samadhi,* which has a number of subtle levels, even the thought disappears and the untroubled, mindless, superconscious state prevails. In this state one experiences a total union where the self seems to merge with everything outside of the self.

To reach these states and hold them takes time, concentration, regular practice, and, in time, a teacher's guidance.

The symbol of samadhi, the union in yoga, is the ajna chakra, the sixth chakra, shown on the next two pages. It is the union of Shiva and his consort Parvati. The union is so consummate that he is shown as the androgyne, half man, half woman, completely fused and balanced, enveloped in the primal sound, the OM, floating in the sky without end, the endless cosmos.

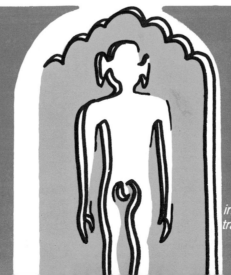

A bronze Jain sculpture of man in Samadhi depicted as a transparent transcendent spirit.

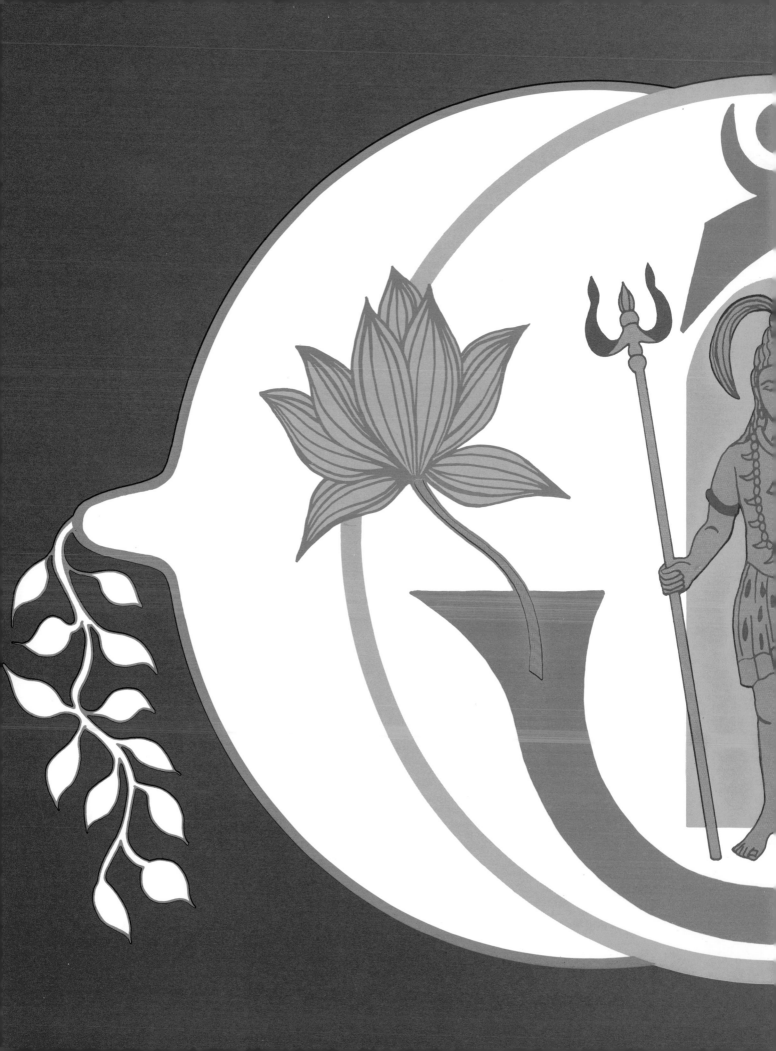

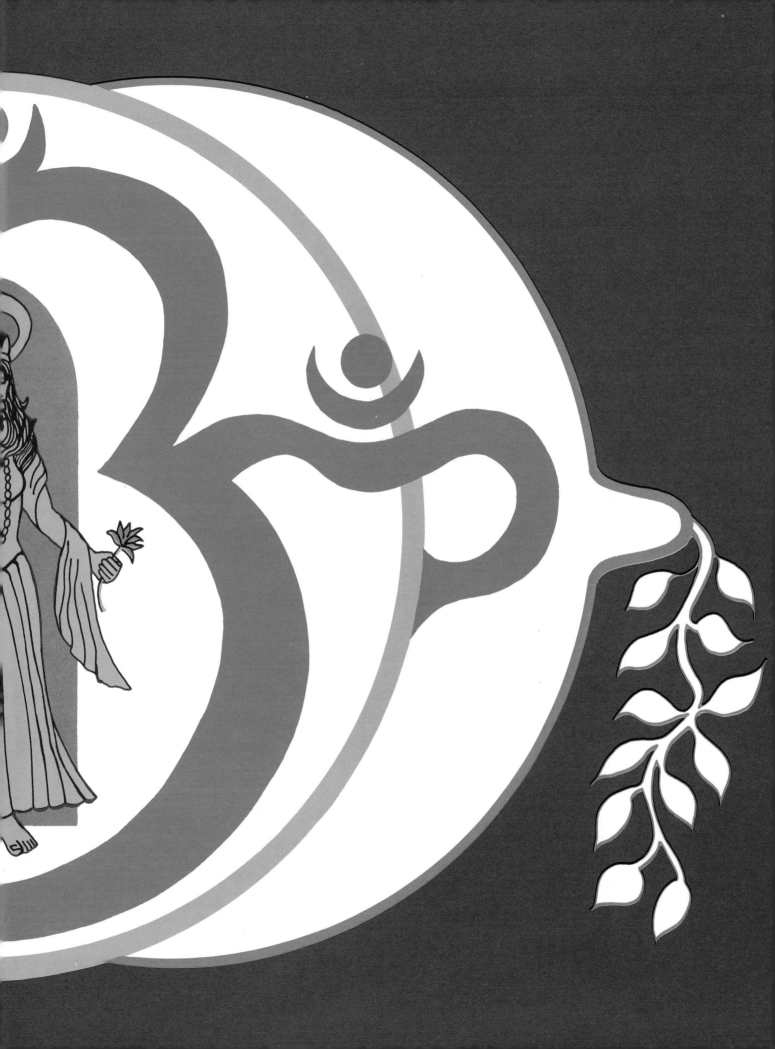

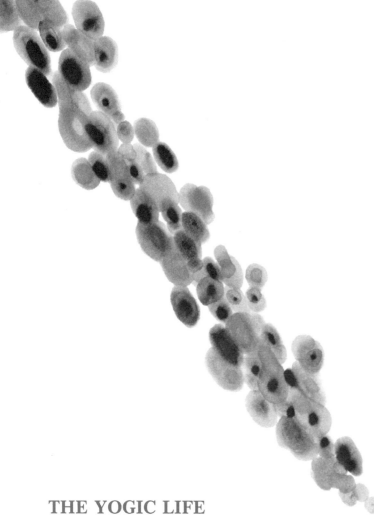

THE YOGIC LIFE

Philosophically, yoga is based on the yamas and niyamas—what in Western terms we would call morals and ethics and the way to try to fulfill them, a kind of ten commandments without the weight of sin.

In writing this section we have tried to be simple, direct, and nondogmatic. These views are only guideposts, short essays on insights we have gained in our lives through Yoga.

The yamas are nonviolence, nonattachment, nonstealing, nonlying and nonlusting. The practices of the niyamas have to do with devotion, austerity, study, cleanliness and contentment.

When we first studied these ideas, they seemed to have a formal quality to us, to be ideals rather than living principles. Working with another gifted teacher whose point of view was slightly different, one more relaxed and Western in context, broadened our insights. The final aims of the yogic life were the same.

The freedom and restlessness that is in the Western psyche has as its positive quality the power to cut through orthodoxy to viable expanded life consciousness.

Yoga starts with the individual as the entity that can be known most profoundly by itself; this self interest is the interest in dynamically developing one's human potentiality. The stress on self could be misconstrued as selfishness. But the self that is striven for is the objective rather than the subjective self.

Yoga is described as skill in action, the skill in bringing into action the understanding of these yamas and niyamas.

Yamas

Nonviolence

Political nonviolence is most familiar to us from the great teachings of Mahatma Gandhi and Martin Luther King. But it is nonviolence to one's own person that is the subtle starting point of understanding this principle.

The student, by doing Hatha Yoga, tries to treat the body well and kindly. His eating and drinking habits nurture rather than harm the body.

In regard to the psyche, self-caused violent action has to do with aggression toward others, mockery, envy, hate and other acts dealing with the yamas and niyamas, like lying and stealing. The feedback as well as the actual experience of any of these acts is violent to one's self.

When you are fully conscious of the concept of nonviolence, you will choose not to violate the self; choice, positive choice, is the key in all yoga discipline and underlies the yamas and niyamas. Often we cannot choose what happens in our lives, but we *can* choose how to deal with these situations so that they feed our inner peace and enjoyment. The choice not to choose can also be a positive prerogative.

It is true that choice can be an illusion. We often operate on subliminal levels which are a mystery to us. The best we can do is to try, creatively, to be in touch with our deepest self. (When that self is fully contacted, choice falls away and one lives unencumbered, in rhythm with another deeper conscious, the intuitive consciousness.)

Through reflection and inner study yoga tries to have one examine this violence and nonviolence, focus in on it and become conscious of it in all the dimensions of daily life.

Nonattachment

Nonattachment to things, to persons, to ideas can sound un-human, irresponsible and austere. Actually the idea is the very opposite. It is living, intense "nowness," full of involvement, feeling, concern and affection.

Nonattachment to people gives them maximum space in which to develop. It guards us from trying to change and shape others. In regard to children and mates this can best be understood by observing that to give learning, support, understanding and compassion without any desire to control is most liberating for their development and ours.

A nonattached person has fresh attitudes to new situations, few preconceived ideas and therefore a nonattachment to expectancy. One who is not attached to goals may still set directions in his life, but the process of getting there is more important than the goal.

Becoming attached to and acquiring things which go beyond our basic needs should always be evaluated by considering what we must do to acquire them, how they enslave our ego and activate our pride.

Materialism is only a point of view toward the material world. If you can readily give up what you own at any time, possessing things is not materialistic.

Nonstealing

Stealing is taking. We easily understand this in regard to physical objects owned by others.

Stealing on a more subtle plane deals with the taking of other people's time, emotions, affections, attentions and moods. Encountering someone when you are in an angry mood and in turn making them feel agitated is to steal that person's mood.

Don't be afraid to use people if you are doing it in a reciprocal way. However, using others to vent your feelings and desires can keep you from developing your innermost strengths and abilities.

Using people's attitudes and ideas, without personal involvement, is really stealing from ourselves the ability to act on our own.

Yoga, through conscious thought, tries to develop this innerdependence and independence.

Nonlying

Honesty is repressed by fear, fear of being oneself, of frankly living and expressing one's feelings.

Nonlying to oneself is a process of scrutiny which keeps us from fooling ourselves and keeps us living without delusion and compensatory posturing. Other people's reactions to our attitudes can also help us to be more insightful.

To exaggerate, distort or lie to others can mean manipulating people for our own ego concerns.

A good way to sharpen our sense of inner truth is to be ready to confess our errors, to be without contrition, yet keenly aware of harm done to others.

To search out truths about ourself on all levels, nonjudgmentally, opens the way for growth. Yoga posits man as a step in the creative evolutionary cycle. Growth through insight is one of the keys to this development.

Nonlusting

Lingering thoughts on one's desires, and not being able to fulfill them, develops excessive attachment to desire. This is the quality of lust.

Desire combined with devotion, love, tenderness and respect joins the act of sexual love to an act of spiritual union.

During lovemaking, climax, and after, the experience of sex can move from sense delight to feelings of complete abandonment of the self, complete fusion with one's mate, complete union with universal forces —a consummation on so many levels that the spiritual aspect of our beings is touched in many profound ways.

Many of the ideas in yoga regarding the sexual life come from the early founders of yoga who were householders. Later, asceticism entered into the Indian religious tradition.

Chastity, especially during the early stages of concentrated yoga practice, is often maintained. This is a way to center and redirect energies. If discipline is thought of as substituting one positive experience for another, then the practice is not a denial.

Living with an intense feeling of union with the cosmos and its most profound truths can be so fulfilling that there is little desire for sex.

Much curiosity exists about Tantric Yoga. To the Tantrist, the female-creative aspect was central to their worship. Basically, Tantric practice dealt with a ritualization of sexual intercourse, so that the mind-set for the sensual experience was connected with the deity and transcendent consciousness.

The refined aspect of this practice involved nonclimaxed sex, where lengthy stimulation produced inner heightening of energy, or where climax was retained within the man's body so that the semen was absorbed.

In the Yoga of the Kundalini, which is part of tantra, strong physical and sexual energies are joined, channeled and directed to give one the experience of spiritual union.

Pure tantra was involved in trying to unify our sex being with our spirit being in a dynamic way.

Niyamas

Devotion

Devotion is love without attachment. It comes when we develop the ability to love and cherish the positivity of another person without the desire to possess him.

Devotional love does not require the return of love. One can give this kind of love in proportion to how good or centered one feels about one's self.

Devotion to the self is self love without pride.

A devotional attitude leads one to live every part of life with a conscious respect for the intrinsic nature of other objects and beings. The self becomes smaller, the understanding larger, and the ability to synchronize with all environments expands.

Devotion to what one calls God, a consciousness which can grow in meditation, is the love, awe and respect for the life process.

Austerity

Austerity, in the yogic sense, could also be defined as simplicity. In regard to material possessions, it discourages acquistion of things one doesn't really need, things which can tie the psyche down. So many of our possessions deal with the past, and the past can weigh heavily on the present.

We often make the mistake, through ownership, of becoming the things we own, of seeing objects as extensions of ourselves.

Simplicity of mind can give us an ability to bring complexity to root essence. In this state, speech becomes more meaningful and less verbose.

Intense concentration on the present keeps preconceived ideas and memories from dominating and filling our present consciousness.

"The head that holds the simple mind has many rooms for God."

Cleanliness

Inner and outer physical cleanliness is basic to yoga; our bodies become purer and lighter when we are clean. There are specific yoga practices to cleanse and purify the body. These, "nettis," are for the advanced student and must be taught personally as they involve the use of strings and cloths to keep nasal passages and stomach areas clean.

Cleanliness can also be thought of as order. Each person's sense of order is different. Because our surroundings often reflect us and affect us, it is important to create a supportive environment.

Aesthetics, the effort of man to bring beauty and enhancement into his physical life, has to do with creative order.

Yoga, through these niyamas and other practices, cleanses the mind and spirit. The clear, ordered mind can see positivity in the most negative situations and can help to clean or clear them up.

Study

The basis for yogic study is concentrated within all the yamas and niyamas. These confront man's involvement with all the life around him and then slowly center in a study of man's inner self.

In meditation one learns by entering the inner self. In study one learns by stepping back and studying the studier.

Study also means a close investigation of books and other media which will inspire and illuminate us. They create an atmosphere of learning around us, voices available at any time to provide the tools and reinforcement we need.

These sources nourish us, feeding us energy as surely as food and water do. In writing this book, those who fed us energy were Gitananda, Vyas Dev, G. Roy, Vishnu Devananda, B. K. S. Iyengar, and Satchidananda.

Reading for enjoyment is different than study (though study for many is enjoyable). The knowledge gained in serious study becomes integrated in our being as an essential resource.

One of our teachers would always end her class by having everyone declare "a respect for the learning process." Study is one of the eight paths of yoga, Gnana Yoga, the path of mind and intellect.

Contentment

Contentment is a state of happiness, happiness arrived at through nonharming action. It is a state of balance and equilibrium, of profound well-being.

Centered activity, which is contented activity, helps one to concentrate and be fully involved in what one is doing so that the action, whatever it may be, is complete. Completed action leaves one with no residue of regret, desire, or guilt.

By accepting that every moment is as it must be, one will not hypothesize that it should have been different. Shoulds, coulds, and ifs lead to a pattern of thinking far from contentment.

To have no desire to know the nature of the next moment is to live without anticipation. Anticipation often leads to disappointment. (At times when anticipation brings anxiety, consciously imagining all possible outcomes can help.) Expectation is wishful and drains energy.

Living in the present moment does not mean that one isn't making future plans. But plans grow more organically from present reality, rather than from dreams and longings, and are more flexible to changes in future reality.

On Food

Basically, we eat to nourish and sustain the body. If man, through greater awareness, can go beyond his taste desires and learned appetites, he can listen to the body's real needs and will spontaneously eat the right foods. Animals have this inherent ability.

According to Indian philosophy, all matter, including food, has one of three qualities—a state of purity, sattva; a state of agitation, rajas; or a state of dullness and inertia, tamas.

In over-cooked, bulky, lifeless food, tamas predominates. When one eats a rajas diet, he chooses food for its spiced, sweet, sour or pickled taste. These foods stimulate rather than nourish and often give a quick, temporary rush of energy. Eating a sattva diet is to reap the direct benefits of food as it exists in nature. Fruits, nuts, fresh picked vegetables, sprouts and whole grains give the body a light yet vital feeling. Your awareness of the inherent qualities of freshness, natural sweetness, tartness, texture and juiciness contained within these foods is sharpened, and you develop a sensitivity to their vital life force.

A yogic diet usually emphasizes sattva, and also contains yogurt, legumes and sometimes eggs and light cheese to give the necessary proteins.

The nutritional value of fruits and vegetables depends upon the quality of the soil in which they are grown. Modern methods of farming often produce fruits and vegetables with inadequate vitamin and mineral content. It is necessary for some people who eat vegetarian diets to use vitamin and mineral supplements.

To be vegetarian does not necessarily make one a spiritual or peaceful person. However, a serious student of yoga does not eat any form of animal life. Meat is hard to digest. It is high in cholesterol and upsets the body's acid–alkaline balance. This fact is now being discovered by Western doctors. It would seem contradictory to build a healthy body through yoga and still eat unhealthy food.

Processed foods containing additives and preservatives can be toxic to the body; refined foods such as white flour, white rice and sugar are highly acid-producing and often cause a mucous condition.

To change your diet radically in a short period of time may harm the body or psyche. One of the things that meat gives to the diet is a certain richness of taste, so when changing over, cook vegetarian dishes which are also rich in taste. There are many.

Our drift toward vegetarianism began while living in Japan. We stopped eating meat, not for any health, humanitarian or religious reasons, but because it seemed to express the way we felt about our life. We did eat some fish. In India, we learned how to eat a completely balanced diet without any animal protein.

In the West, vegetarianism is a growing life style. There is much information available in books, magazines and media, as well as products in stores, to help you to eat in a more healthy, natural and yogic way.

On Fasting

To fast one day each week can be a healthy thing. It gives the digestive system a day of rest. Be sure, when you try it, to drink plenty of water on that day. It will help to cleanse the system, and make up for the liquid you are missing from the food you usually eat.

By fasting, we come to realize that we eat more than we need and that, with a little practice, we can control the urgency to eat at will. It is part of the discipline of controlling the body rather than having it control us.

If you feel a pang of hunger during your fast, try to relax; concentrate on whatever you are doing and the desire for food will pass. Rather than making you feel weak, fasting can build energy, for the body is not working at assimilating the food.

Fasting can be an aid to meditation by acting to quiet the body's appetite and allowing the concentration to be put entirely on the mind.

The curative power of fasting is known to be effective in many illnesses.

Three to four days is a good period for an extended fast. The meals leading up to a fast should be light. An enema should be taken on the third day to cleanse out the wastes which are still being eliminated. When breaking the fast, eat meals of bland, cooked vegetables. Slowly, taking a few days, return to the raw and roughage foods.

Fasts of longer than four days should be done under knowledgeable supervision, both in regard to the psyche and the body. Longer fasts, though there can be some temporary feelings of weakness, give one a great sense of well being, and one's awareness of many things is sharpened at these times. Very lengthy periods of fasting can cause trance states which may or may not be of value to one's personal growth. These should be taken under supervision.

Fasting to do penance is *not* part of the yogic attitude towards life.

On Silence, Fasting of Words

To be in silence for a day or longer is like fasting, the building into the self of a new rhythm which can have very positive and revealing results.

In India, there are two kinds of practices of silence, one where a blackboard or paper is used to communicate and another where all communication is avoided.

By not talking, your mind takes a whole inward direction; a strong feeling of containment usually comes at this time.

By getting out of the usual pattern of listening and responding, the mind quiets and only listens. Your perception of what people are saying around you increases amazingly; the mind is not busy thinking up responses. You start to hear the person behind and beyond the words.

Not talking removes one of our ego functions. The quiet of silence puts us more in the rhythm of the universe around us.

A famous contemporary teacher in India, Meher Baba, was silent for 44 years. Buckminster Fuller, the revolutionary American architect and philospher, chose to be silent for 1 year at a crisis time in his early life.

Silence combined with a day of fasting can provide a powerful psychic cleansing.

On Laughing

Laughter on a vibrational level is an explosion of high energy electrical pulsars, coming in rounds, rising and falling, releasing energy. It is an exterior manifestation of intense energies that are felt internally in high meditative experience. "Laughter is divine." It is one of our most direct expressions of happiness and joy.

An Indian friend, when he felt amused, happy, or just wanted to raise the group psyche, would direct his attention to one of the people in our group and start to laugh. It would immediately become infectious and spread. To search for what was funny was to miss the point—anything became a source of amusement, especially those who could not abandon themselves to the laughter. It could go on for hours (our friend believed it was excellent for the digestion after meals).

The group interplay of laughter, like the interplay of improvised sound (page 109), is a very elevated thing, pure, without any stimulation except the building laughter itself.

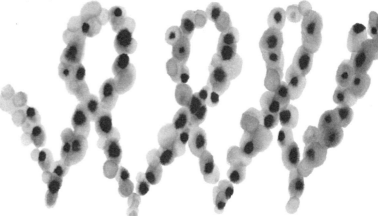

We are all receptors and sources of untapped power.

Living the yamas and niyamas gives one strength, understanding, and power. This power is not dominating but loving in spirit.

Power helps us to transcend our difficulties. Rather than feeling victimized by our misfortunes, we can use them as challenges to our power.

Transcending these challenges releases new energy and power.

This spiraling release of energies brings us to an opening of our intuitive and spiritual power.